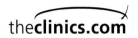
theclinics.com

SLEEP MEDICINE CLINICS

Sleep-Related Breathing Disorders and Positive Airway Pressure Therapy in Adults

Guest Editors
MAX HIRSHKOWITZ, PhD, D ABSM
AMIR SHARAFKHANEH, MD, D ABSM

December 2006 • Volume 1 • Number 4

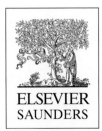

ELSEVIER
SAUNDERS

An imprint of Elsevier, Inc
PHILADELPHIA LONDON TORONTO MONTREAL SYDNEY TOKYO

W.B. SAUNDERS COMPANY
A Division of Elsevier Inc.

1600 John F. Kennedy Boulevard • Suite 1800 • Philadelphia, PA 19103-2899

http://www.sleep.theclinics.com

SLEEP MEDICINE CLINICS Volume 1, Number 4
December 2006 ISSN 1556-407X, ISBN 1-4160-3922-8

Editor: Sarah E. Barth

The ideas and opinions expressed in *Sleep Medicine Clinics* do not necessarily reflect those of the Publisher. The Publisher does not assume any responsibility for any injury and/or damage to persons or property arising out of or related to any use of the material contained in this periodical. The reader is advised to check the appropriate medical literature and the product information currently provided by the manufacturer of each drug to be administered to verify the dosage, the method and duration of administration, or contraindications. It is the responsibility of the treating physician or other health care professional, relying on independent experience and knowledge of the patient, to determine drug dosages and the best treatment for the patient. Mention of any product in this issue should not be construed as endorsement by the contributors, editors, or the Publisher of the product or manufacturers' claims.

Sleep Medicine Clinics (ISSN 1556-407X) is published quarterly by W.B. Saunders Company, 360 Park Avenue South, New York, NY 10010-1710. Months of publication are March, June, September and December. Business and editorial offices: 1600 John F. Kennedy Boulevard, Suite 1800, Philadelphia, PA 19103-2899. Accounting and circulation offices: 6277 Sea Harbor Drive, Orlando, FL 32887-4800. Periodicals postage paid at New York, and additional mailing offices. Subscription prices are $129.00 per year (US individuals), $50.00 (US students), $259.00 (US institutions), $149.00 (Canadian individuals), $85.00 (Canadian and foreign students), $279.00 (Canadian institutions), $149.00 (foreign individuals), and $279.00 (foreign institutions). Foreign air speed delivery is included in all *Clinics* subscription prices. All prices are subject to change without notice. POSTMASTER: Send address changes to *Sleep Medicine Clinics*, Elsevier Periodicals Customer Service, 6277 Sea Harbor Drive, FL 32887-4800. **Customer Service: 1-800-654-2452 (US). From outside of the United States, call 1-407-345-4000. E-mail: hhspcs@wbsaunders.com**.

Reprints: For copies of 100 or more, of articles in this publication, please contact the Commercial Reprints Department, Elsevier Inc., 360 Park Avenue South, New York, New York 10010-1710. Tel.: (212) 633-3813, Fax: (212) 462-1935, e-mail: reprints@elsevier.com

Printed in the United States of America.

SLEEP-RELATED BREATHING DISORDERS AND POSITIVE AIRWAY PRESSURE THERAPY IN ADULTS

CONSULTING EDITOR

TEOFILO LEE-CHIONG, JR., MD
Head, Section of Sleep Medicine, National Jewish
Medical and Research Center, Denver; Associate
Professor of Medicine, University of Colorado
Health Sciences Center, Denver, Colorado

GUEST EDITORS

MAX HIRSHKOWITZ, PhD, D ABSM
Tenured Associate Professor, Baylor College of
Medicine, Department of Medicine and
Department of Psychiatry, Houston; Michael E.
DeBakey Veterans Affairs Medical Center,
Houston, Texas

AMIR SHARAFKHANEH, MD, D ABSM
Assistant Professor of Medicine and Director, Sleep
Medicine Fellowship Program, Baylor College of
Medicine, Houston, Texas; Medical Director, Sleep
Disorders and Research Center, Michael E.
DeBakey Veterans Affairs Medical Center,
Houston, Texas

CONTRIBUTORS

AGOSTINHO DA ROSA, PhD
Stanford University Sleep Medicine Program and
Biomedical Engineering Laboratory of
the University of Lisbon (Lisbon), Stanford,
California

HEIDEMARIE GAST, MD
Sleep Disorders and Research Center,
Michael E. DeBakey Veterans Affairs Medical
Center, Houston; Baylor College
of Medicine, Houston, Texas; Department of
Neurology, Universität Witten/Herdecke,
Witten, Germany

NILGUN GIRAY, MD
Assistant Professor, Department of Psychiatry,
Baylor College of Medicine, Houston, Texas

SHEILA GOODNIGHT-WHITE, MD
Professor of Medicine, Baylor College
of Medicine, Houston; Section Chief,
Pulmonary, Critical Care and Sleep Medicine
Section, Michael E. DeBakey Veterans Affairs
Medical Center, Houston, Texas

CHRISTIAN GUILLEMINAULT, MD, BIOLD
Stanford University Sleep Medicine Program,
Stanford, California

CHAD C. HAGEN, MD
Stanford University Sleep Medicine Program,
Stanford, California

ALI M. HASHMI, MD
Research Associate, Michael E. DeBakey Veterans
Affairs Medical Center, Sleep Disorders Center,
Houston, Texas

MAX HIRSHKOWITZ, PhD, D ABSM
Tenured Associate Professor, Baylor College
of Medicine, Department of Medicine and
Department of Psychiatry, Houston; Michael E.
DeBakey Veterans Affairs Medical Center,
Houston, Texas

JOHANNES JÖRG, MD
Department of Neurology, Universität Witten/
Herdecke, Witten, Germany

MEIR KRYGER, MD, Saint Boniface General
Hospital Sleep Laboratory & University of
Manitoba, Winnipeg, Canada

CHARLIE K. LAN, DO, D ABSM
Assistant Professor of Medicine, Baylor College of
Medicine, Houston; Michael E. DeBakey Veterans
Affairs Medical Center, Houston, Texas

TEOFILO LEE-CHIONG, JR., MD
Head, Section of Sleep Medicine, National
Jewish Medical and Research Center, Denver;
Associate Professor of Medicine, University
of Colorado Health Sciences Center,
Denver, Colorado

MICHAEL LITTNER, MD
Section Chief, Pulmonary and Critical Care
Medicine, Veterans Administration Medical
Center, Sepulveda, California

OLGA PRILIPKO, MD
Stanford University Sleep Medicine Program,
Stanford, California

HUBERT RINGENDAHL, MD
Department of Neurology, Universität
Witten/Herdecke, Witten, Germany

MARY W. ROSE, PsyD, CBSM
Assistant Professor of Medicine, Baylor College of
Medicine, Houston; Michael E. DeBakey Veterans
Affairs Medical Center, Houston, Texas

SUSANNE SCHWALEN, MD
Department of Neurology, Universität Witten/
Herdecke, Witten, Germany

AMIR SHARAFKHANEH, MD, D ABSM
Assistant Professor of Medicine and Director, Sleep
Medicine Fellowship Program, Baylor College of
Medicine, Houston, Texas; Medical Director, Sleep
Disorders and Research Center, Michael E.
DeBakey Veterans Affairs Medical Center,
Houston, Texas

HOSSEIN SHARAFKHANEH, MD
Research Assistant, Section of Pulmonary, Critical
Care and Sleep Medicine, Baylor College of
Medicine, Houston, Texas

NIZAR SULEMAN, MD
Baylor College of Medicine, Department of
Medicine, Houston, Texas

SURYAKANTA VELAMURI, MD
Assistant Professor, Sleep Disorders and Research
Center, Michael E. DeBakey Veterans Affairs
Medical Center, Houston; Baylor College of
Medicine, Houston, Texas

TERRY YOUNG, PhD
Professor, Department Population Health
Sciences, School of Medicine and Public Health,
University of Wisconsin, Madison, Madison,
Wisconsin

SLEEP-RELATED BREATHING DISORDERS AND POSITIVE AIRWAY PRESSURE THERAPY IN ADULTS

Volume 1 • Number 4 • December 2006

Contents

Diagnosed sleep apnea is common (2.9%) among Veterans Health Administration (VHA) beneficiaries. The projected actuarial prevalence may be 16% or more when extrapolated from published data. Further studies are needed to establish the true prevalence of sleep apnea in this population. Accurate information is required for appropriate resource allocation to meet health care needs of VHA beneficiaries. Importantly, strong associations between cardiovascular and other conditions and diagnosed sleep apnea were found, extending previously reported findings to the VHA beneficiary population. While the causal role of sleep apnea in these conditions cannot be determined from these data, the authors' findings stress the need for further studies. Understanding the impact of increased case-finding and therapeutic interventions for sleep apnea on patient outcomes, health care utilization, and cost in this high-risk population remains a high priority.

Clinical assessment of a patient who has sleep-related breathing disorders (SRBD) begins with a comprehensive interview. This clinical interview helps identify signs and symptoms, establishes the patient's routine sleep–wake schedule, helps the provider make a proper differential diagnosis, and prompts ordering relevant diagnostic tests. This article illustrates a comprehensive overview of patient interviews and questionnaires, and provides detailed information on laboratory assessment to effectively guide treatment of SRBD.

Portable monitoring systems designed for nonlaboratory assessment of sleep-related breathing disorders are another tool available for practicing sleep medicine. Many of these level III devices are sleep cardiopulmonary recorders. These devices are not intended to replace polysomnography, but rather to complement it when appropriate. When properly integrated into a sleep disorders program, nonlaboratory assessment can facilitate diagnosis of patients who have more severe sleep-disordered breathing.

This study shows that the cost of studies to diagnose obstructive sleep apnea (OSA) can be modeled. When cardiopulmonary recording (CPR) is used as a tool to diagnose OSA in populations in different practice settings, a cost savings-excess amount can be projected based on the cost of polysomnography (PSG), CPR:PSG cost ratio, as well as the proportion of patients with an apnea plus hypopnea index 15 to 30 (category B) in the populations. CPR at its current cost does not provide a cost-effective means to diagnose OSA; however, cost savings can be achieved if the cost of CPR is lower than 10–20% the cost of PSG.

Upper airway resistance syndrome is an important variant in the spectrum of sleep-related breathing disorders. Although not as obvious as sleep apnea in terms of pathophysiology, symptoms, and diagnosis, it frequently is the cause of excessive daytime sleepiness, fatigue, and other long-term sequelae. Further research is required on all aspects of this disorder to improve the understanding and provide appropriate patient care.

There is poor correlation between daytime complaints of patients with sleep disordered breathing and visual scoring of sleep disruption. Cyclic Alternating Pattern (CAP) brings new information on nonrapid eye movement sleep disturbances. An automatic scoring of CAP based on one central EEG lead was developed. Testing of the automatic analytic program by members of the CAP consensus group was performed. The summary of the different steps of the validation of the program, and Mutual Agreement findings between different scorers performing visual scoring and automatic scoring are summarized. An application of the scoring program was done on polysomnograms of young women with sleep complaints compared to non-complaining–matched control women.

A prospective, randomized, parallel control group outcome trial comparing improvement from baseline at 2-week follow-up in treated versus untreated groups was conducted to assess continuous positive airway pressure (CPAP)-related changes in sleepiness in patients with obstructive sleep apnea (OSA). In addition to reduced self-reported sleepiness, CPAP therapy also improved electroencephalographically indexed sleepiness (MWT) in patients with OSA. Not surprisingly, patients who strictly adhered to therapeutic regimen showed the most improvement.

commonly prescribed. Further studies are needed to assess the benefits of CPAP therapy for patients who have less severe OSA and to specify better the positive cardiovascular outcomes.

Mary W. Rose

Positive airway pressure therapy is the optimal treatment for the overwhelming majority of patients who have obstructive sleep apnea, and the American Academy of Sleep Medicine Practice Parameters notes that continuous positive airway pressure (CPAP) is the first-line treatment for severe apnea. Despite the significant benefits of CPAP use, a significant proportion of patients are unable or unwilling to adhere to treatment. This article discusses ways of identifying patients likely to be noncompliant and ways to help them adjust to CPAP treatment.

Charlie K. Lan and Mary W. Rose

Obstructive sleep apnea (OSA) is a prevalent disease, and many patients who undergo surgery suffer from OSA. Because OSA increases the risk of perioperative complications, preoperative evaluation should include assessment for the presence of OSA and the adequacy of OSA therapy. Optimization of OSA therapy preoperatively may reduce perioperative complications related to OSA. Ultimately, a well-developed protocol for perioperative evaluation and management of patients who have OSA may reduce perioperative complications in these patients.

SLEEP MEDICINE CLINICS

Sleep Med Clin 1 (2006) xi–xii

Foreword

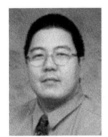

Teofilo Lee-Chiong, Jr., MD
National Jewish Medical and Research Center
1400 Jackson Street, Room J232
Denver, CO 80206, USA

E-mail address:
Lee-Chiongt@njc.org

Teofilo Lee-Chiong, Jr., MD
Consulting Editor

Several conditions can cause respiratory abnormalities during sleep, including obstructive sleep apnea (OSA) syndrome, in which inadequate ventilation occurs despite continued efforts to breath, resulting from upper airway obstruction, central sleep apnea syndrome (absent or diminished respiratory effort), or chronic alveolar hypoventilation syndromes with sleep-related hypercapnia.

OSA is estimated to affect about 24% of males aged 30 to 60 years and 9% of similarly aged females if the disorder is defined by the presence of an apnea–hypopnea index (AHI) of 5 or more. Prevalence of OSA is affected by age, gender, body morphology, weight, race, and medication use. Several factors influence the clinical severity of OSA, namely the AHI, degree of daytime sleepiness and functional impairment, nadir of oxygen saturation, extent of sleep fragmentation, presence of nocturnal arrhythmias related to respiratory events, and presence of co-morbid disorders such as ischemic heart disease or congestive heart failure. Clinical manifestations that should alert the clinician to the possibility of OSA include complaints of snoring, accounts of witnessed apneas, repeated awakenings with gasping or choking,

nighttime diaphoresis, morning headaches, nocturia, and alterations in mood. Daytime sleepiness is a common complaint; however, the absence of daytime sleepiness does not exclude the presence of this disorder. OSA has been associated with greater mortality and significant adverse cardiovascular, psychiatric, and social consequences. By impairing vigilance and increasing sleepiness, it increases driving- and work-related accident rates and impairs neurocognitive function and performance.

Polysomnography is required for the diagnosis of OSA, because clinical and physical examination features are neither sufficiently sensitive nor specific for this disorder. Goals of therapy for OSA include improving sleep quality, relieving daytime symptoms such as excessive sleepiness, enhancing quality of life, and preventing long-term neurocognitive and cardiovascular consequences of untreated or partially treated sleep apnea. A variety of therapies for OSA have been described, including general measures such as avoidance of alcohol and muscle relaxants, weight reduction for patients who are overweight, positional therapy for those whose apnea occurs exclusively or predominantly during

doi:10.1016/j.jsmc.2006.12.003

a supine sleep position, oxygen supplementation, pharmacotherapy, positive airway pressure (PAP) therapy, oral devices, or upper airway surgery.

PAP therapy is the treatment of choice for most patients with OSA and has salutary effects on mortality, cardiovascular profiles, daytime alertness, neurocognitive function, mood, sleep quality, and health care use. Continuous positive airway pressure (CPAP) is very effective in symptomatic patients with moderate and severe OSA, and the beneficial effects of CPAP are sustained over time. However, less than optimal CPAP use is a significant problem in clinical practice. Oral devices worn during sleep may be considered for snorers and individuals with mild to moderate OSA who are intolerant of PAP therapy, or whose OSA persists following upper airway surgery. Upper airway surgery may be considered in patients who are either unwilling or unable to use positive airway pressure therapy. Surgical procedures may be particularly useful for patients with definitive craniofacial or upper airway abnormalities. Finally, modafinil, a wake-promoting agent, may be considered as an adjunct therapy for improving alertness and wakefulness in patients with residual daytime sleepiness despite optimal nasal CPAP therapy for OSA.

Upper airway resistance syndrome (UARS) is a term that has been used to describe a pattern of repetitive sleep-related episodes of increasing resistance in the upper airways with a decrease in inspiratory airflow, increased or constant respiratory effort and arousals from sleep (referred to as respiratory effort–related arousals). In patients with UARS, the AHI is less than 5 events per hour, and there is no accompanying oxygen desaturation. Snoring may or may not be present. Frequent arousals associated with UARS can result in sleep fragmentation. Affected individuals often complain of excessive sleepiness and fatigue.

Central sleep apnea is characterized by repetitive apneic episodes during sleep without associated ventilatory efforts. Central sleep apnea is estimated to represent about 5% to 10% of patients with sleep-related breathing disorders. It can result either from a failure of ventilatory drive (idiopathic form) or from secondary causes such as congestive heart failure or neurological disorders. The idiopathic form is less common than secondary causes. Central apneas can also occur during sleep onset in otherwise healthy individuals and during sleep at high altitude. Therapy, including oxygen supplementation, PAP, or use of pharmacologic agents, varies depending on whether the patient has idiopathic or secondary CSA, or hypercapnic or nonhypercapnic forms of CSA.

Drs. Max Hirshkowitz and Amir Sharafkhaneh have, in this issue, gathered several internationally renowned authorities in the area of sleep-related breathing disorders, who have each provided a current and concise overview of the many aspects of sleep apnea. Readers will appreciate the carefully written discussions on this highly complex field of sleep medicine.

SLEEP
MEDICINE
CLINICS

Sleep Med Clin 1 (2006) xiii–xiv

Preface

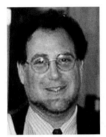 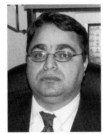

Max Hirshkowitz,
PhD, D ABSM

Amir Sharafkhaneh,
MD, D ABSM

Guest Editors

Max Hirshkowitz, PhD, D ABSM
MED VAMC Sleep Center
2002 Holcombe Boulevard
Houston, TX 77030, USA

E-mail address:
maxh@bcm.tmc.edu

Amir Sharafkhaneh, MD, D ABSM
MED VAMC Sleep Center
2002 Holcombe Boulevard
Houston, TX 77030, USA

E-mail address:
amirs@bcm.tmc.edu

Thirty years ago, sleep-related breathing disorders (SRBDs) were barely on the radar of mainstream medicine. There was some general acknowledgment of hypoventilation in the fanciful dubbing of sleepy, red-faced, morbidly obese individuals as victims of "Pickwickian Syndrome," after Charles Dickens's fictional character "Joe, the fat boy." Although a Kroc Foundation–sponsored conference about sleep apnea was held in California in 1977 and its proceedings were published the following year, SRBDs remained within the domain of a very small group of sleep disorders specialists. Things have changed! Sleep medicine is now a recognized medical specialty with fellowship training programs accredited by the Accreditation Council for Graduate Medical Education. At the forefront of sleep medicine are SRBDs, which are also the driving economic force behind the proliferation of sleep laboratories in virtually every city across the country. If you search "sleep apnea" using PubMed, the system reports almost 15,000 citations published in the indexed medical journals. A search today showed 86 citations in the New England Journal of Medicine, which is currently enjoying a lively debate about SRBD's relationship to heart disease and stroke. Sleep may indeed be "a new cardiovascular frontier" as hailed by Virend Somers.

In this issue, we have put together a mix of articles. Some articles review basic information concerning methods and treatments designed to inform and educate clinicians. We cover clinical, laboratory, and nonlaboratory assessment techniques, as well as positive airway pressure, the standard therapeutic approach. Other articles present literature reviews to provide the reader both classic knowledge and information about recent developments. We are also pleased to be able to include several articles presenting new investigational data. These research studies focus on SRBD's association with other diseases, functions, or sleep phenomena.

Epidemiological studies consistently reinforce the now well-established SRBD prevalence rates.

Some of these studies provide data concerning occurrence in specific and high-risk populations. The first article in this issue reviews epidemiological literature and includes some additional information derived from the Veterans Health Administration inpatient and outpatient databases. The risk for hypertension, diabetes, heart failure, cardiovascular disease, and cerebrovascular disease are tabulated for this population. The second article discusses clinical and laboratory methodologies used to assess SRBD. In the past decade, measurements, definitions, and metrics have evolved. Some ambiguities have been resolved, but others remain. Some of our metrics are based on qualitative measures and others on quantitative measures. Also, surrogate measurements are commonly used. Thus, it is important that clinicians grasp the underlying mechanism of measurement technique to properly appreciate the meaning of our clinical diagnostic and treatment outcome measures.

The current diagnostic standard for SRBD involves recording electroencephalography, electrooculography, electromyography, airflow, respiratory effort, heart rhythm, oximetry, and leg movements continuously, all night, in a sleep laboratory, with a technologist present. This procedure is called attended polysomnography and it is thorough but expensive. SRBD, especially in fairly severe cases, can be detected using cardiopulmonary recorders that monitor airflow, respiratory effort, heart rhythm, and oximetry. How best to use this new technology is hotly debated. Proponents on one side advocate in favor of overnight cardiopulmonary recording, touting its ease, lower cost, and practicality. Other sleep experts seem dead set against abbreviated home recording systems. When listening to these debates, one gets the impression that "east is east and west is west and never the twain shall meet." Nonetheless, in this issue, we have included a brief article that describes an approach using both laboratory and home methods in a complementary fashion within a sleep program. Furthermore, this approach is actually in use and functions well. To complement the description of this hybrid approach, we included an article describing how to assess portable monitor use to determine its economic advantage or disadvantage in different populations.

The next two articles describe newer frontiers in SRBD. The first reviews and describes upper airway resistance syndrome and the next analyzes sleep instability indexed with cyclic alternating pattern in young women with sleep-disordered breathing. Research findings unpublished until now concerning the relationship between SRBD and sleepiness, cognition, and mood are presented in the three articles that follow. These data are consistent with and extend existing knowledge about SRBD alterations of neurobehavioral phenomena. A review aricle follows, addressing quality-of-life issues.

Positive airway pressure is standard therapy for SRBD, and the final three articles describe its different forms, issues relating to therapeutic adherence, and use in peri-operative management of patients with SRBD. Although other treatment modalities exist, the scope of this issue considers only positive pressure intervention. An entire volume could easily and at some point in the future probably will be dedicated entirely to orthodontic, surgical, medical, weight-loss, and the variety of positive pressure treatment approaches for SRBD.

Our understanding of SRBDs has dramatically improved in the past decade. Moreover, the clinical community now appreciates SRBD's importance. In closing, we wish to express our appreciation for the efforts of our colleagues who contributed to this volume, to the vast army of researchers and clinicians who daily advance the field, and our subjects in research studies who consent to being poked, prodded, questioned, and examined so that we may better measure, correlate, and understand the wide spectrum of SRBDs.

SLEEP
MEDICINE
CLINICS

Sleep Med Clin 1 (2006) 443–447

Epidemiology of Sleep-Related Breathing Disorders: Comparisons with the Veterans Health Administration Databases

Amir Sharafkhaneh, MD, D ABSM[a,b,*],
Sheila Goodnight White, MD[a,b], Hossein Sharafkhaneh, MD[a,b],
Max Hirshkowitz, PhD, D ABSM[a,b], Terry Young, PhD[c,d]

Symptomatic obstructive sleep apnea (OSA) afflicts an estimated 4% of men and 2% of women between the ages of 30 and 70 years [1]. OSA is characterized by repeated pharyngeal obstructions during sleep causing airflow cessation (apnea) or reduction (hypopnea). OSA events produce arousals and fragment sleep and often are accompanied by oxygen desaturations. Common symptoms include daytime sleepiness, fatigue, irritability, disturbed sleep, memory problems, and diminished quality of life [2,3]. Recent epidemiologic studies link untreated OSA with hypertension, heart disease, stroke, and increased risk for motor vehicle accidents [4–8]. Although OSA epidemiology is well studied in the general population [9], data from high-risk populations are limited. Risk factors and

comorbidities associated with OSA are common among Veterans Health Administration (VHA) beneficiaries; therefore, the authors expected to find a high prevalence. Only few small studies in this high-risk population have been reported, however. Ancoli-Israel and colleagues [10], in a study of inpatient VHA beneficiaries 65 to 91 years old, reported a sleep apnea (apnea index > 5) prevalence of 36%. Similarly, Kreis and colleagues [11], in a study of VHA beneficiaries, reported a 27% prevalence of sleep apnea (7 of 26) when sleep apnea was defined as more than 30 episodes of apnea per night. Similar prevalence is reported for the outpatient setting. Ancoli-Israel and colleagues [12] studied 117 subjects referred to their outpatient sleep clinic at a Veterans Administration Medical Center. Fifty-one

This work is supported in part by the Office of Research & Development of Department of Veterans Affairs.
a Baylor College of Medicine, 1 Baylor Plaza, Houston, TX 77030, USA
b Sleep Disorders & Research Center, Michael E. DeBakey Veterans Affairs Medical Center (111i), 2002 Holcombe Blvd., Houston, TX 77030, USA
c University of Wisconsin School of Medicine, Madison, WI 53706, USA
d US Department of Public Health, Madison, WI 53703, USA
* Corresponding author. Sleep Center (111i), 2002 Holcombe Blvd., Houston, TX 77030.
E-mail address: amirs@bcm.tmc.edu (A. Sharafkhaneh).

doi:10.1016/j.jsmc.2006.10.002

patients (44%) had sleep apnea as defined by 30 or more apneic events for the study night.

Veterans Health Administration databases

The VHA provides health care to more than 4 million veterans. In 1970, the VHA began developing centralized databases to monitor the care provided and to store related information for each inpatient or outpatient visit. Access to these databases is available for research. These databases have been used previously for study of different diseases. Recently investigators from the Houston VA Medical Centers Health Services Research and Development used these databases to report hospital use and survival among VHA beneficiaries [13].

The databases include the Patient Treatment File (PTF) and the Outpatient File (OPC). Each annual PTF file contains approximately 0.5 million hospitalization records among more than 300,000 United States military veterans. The PTF was established in 1970 and registers all hospitalizations from 172 VA hospitals throughout the United States. Diagnoses recorded by practitioners at each VHA facility are entered by trained coders into the local computer system and then are transferred automatically to the central VA database in Austin, Texas. Each hospitalization has a primary discharge diagnosis and up to nine secondary diagnoses, encoded according to the ninth revision of the Clinical Modification of the International Classification of Diseases. In contrast, the OPC contains information concerning outpatient clinic visits. In 1997 the VHA began recording the OPC diagnoses made during each outpatient encounter. With the use of unique identifiers (social security numbers), an individual can be tracked through the different files of the PTF and OPC to obtain a complete record of encounters in the system.

Veterans Health Administration database results

We performed a retrospective, cross-sectional, database review of all VHA Outpatient Clinic Files (OCF) and Patient Treatment Files (PTF) from the beginning of fiscal year 1998 to the end of fiscal year 2001. We searched the VA's inpatient hospitalization (PTF) and outpatient clinic visit (OPC) database files for the appearance of ICD-9-CM diagnosis codes for sleep apnea, including: insomnia with sleep apnea (780.51); hypersomnia with sleep apnea (780.53); and other unspecified sleep apnea (780.57). The database showed 146,548 patients identified with these codes during the fiscal years from 1992–2001 (1992–2001 for PTF and 1997–2001 for OPC). In this study, almost 3% of

VHA beneficiaries were found to carry a diagnosis of sleep apnea [14]. However, it is important to stress that the 2.9% prevalence in that study was only for clinically diagnosed sleep apnea. To estimate the overall prevalence of sleep apnea in the authors' population, the authors used published data from Young and colleagues [15]. In mailed questionnaire administered to 4925 working adult men and women, only 14 men and two women reported that they had been told by a doctor that they had sleep apnea. For the male cohort, a prevalence of clinically diagnosed sleep apnea of 0.62% was reported. Subsequently, 1090 of this cohort underwent overnight polysomnography protocol [1]. Moderate-to-severe screen-detected sleep apnea syndrome (SAS) was defined as daytime sleepiness and an apnea/hypopnea index (AHI) of 15 or higher. Seventy-seven male subjects met the definition for moderate-to-severe SAS. The authors concluded that only 14 of the 77 men (18%) who met the criteria for moderate-to-severe SAS were clinically diagnosed before the screening. Using the formula, 100% − % (clinically diagnosed SAS/screen-detected SAS), they estimated that 82% [100% − % (14/77)] of men who have moderate-to-severe SAS are undiagnosed. Although the population in Young's study [15] is different from that in the authors' study, the findings indicate that 2.9% is an underestimate of sleep apnea prevalence in VHA beneficiaries. Accordingly, the 118,105 subjects who have diagnosed sleep apnea may account for up to only 18% of the total sleep apnea cohort in the authors' study population. Therefore, the likely total number of persons who have sleep apnea may be as high as 656,138 (118,105 × 100/18). With this number, a prevalence of 16% (656,138/4,060,504) is likely. If confirmed, this information is important for planning resource allocation. Furthermore, the number of the newly diagnosed cases increased during the study period. This change probably reflects increasing awareness of sleep apnea among practitioners, establishment of sleep apnea–related guidelines within the VHA, and the availability of sleep facilities and professionals.

Data comparisons

The estimated prevalence of 16% is in sharp contrast with the 4% prevalence of sleep apnea in the general population reported by Young and colleagues [1] in their well-designed prospective study. This difference presumably relates to a higher prevalence of sleep apnea risk factors in the authors' population. Alternatively, the higher prevalence of diagnosed sleep apnea among VHA beneficiaries may result from greater self-selection and referral bias: patients who interface with the health care system more frequently are more likely to obtain diagnoses, including sleep apnea and comorbid conditions diagnoses.

Although the mean age for patients who had sleep apnea in the authors' population was comparable with other studies, age distribution differed [16–18]. The prevalence of diagnosed sleep apnea was 1.76% in the age range of 35 to 64 years and was 1.38% for patients aged 65 years and older. By contrast, studies that prospectively define OSA with polysomnography show increased OSA prevalence as a function of age. This difference may arise from case definition. Generally, OSA in older individuals is characterized by more central events and less-severe disease. Bixler and colleagues [16] found that although polysomnographically diagnosed OSA is more common in older individuals, the prevalence of symptomatic OSA (defined as an AHI $\geq$ 10 with symptoms) is lower (4.7% for age < 65 years, versus 1.7% for age $\geq$ 65 years). Furthermore, notwithstanding the higher prevalence of OSA in elders, most of the increase in OSA prevalence occurs before age 65 years [16,19–21]. By contrast, the authors' study included only symptomatic patients who were referred for evaluation on the basis of clinical suspicion and who subsequently were diagnosed as having sleep apnea.

Comorbidities

As expected, the authors found a strong association between diagnosed obesity and diabetes mellitus with sleep apnea; this finding is consistent with published literature [22–25]. Diabetes mellitus is a common complication of obesity [26]. Prevalence for diagnosed obesity and diabetes mellitus were similar among individuals who had sleep apnea; however, in subjects who have diagnosed sleep apnea the odds ratio for diagnosed obesity is more than twice that for diagnosed diabetes mellitus. This pattern probably

derives from more consistent criteria and greater sensitivity for diabetes mellitus than for obesity. Clinical criteria for obesity tend to be less sensitive (and often are based on clinical judgment rather than body mass index). Thus, patients classified as obese are more likely to be extreme cases. These classification differences can introduce differential bias.

The authors' data revealed a high association between diagnosed cardiovascular comorbid conditions and diagnosed sleep apnea (Table 1). The odds ratios—adjusted for age, gender, and ethnicity—for these comorbid conditions with sleep apnea were strong and statistically significant; because our sample was large (n = 98,735), the 95% confidence intervals were narrow (all p<0.0001). Not surprisingly, the association between sleep apnea and hypertension was strong. This association is consistent with published cross-sectional and prospective studies [6,17,27–30].

As is presented in Table 1, diagnosed cardiovascular disease is common in VHA beneficiaries diagnosed as having sleep apnea. This relationship is supported by other observational studies. For example, in the Sleep Heart Health study, Shahar and colleagues [31] reported 42% greater odds of prevalent coronary heart disease in individuals who had an AHI of more than 11 events per hour of sleep than in individuals who had an AHI of fewer than 1.3 events per hour of sleep. They also found a high prevalence of diagnosed heart failure in the authors' population. In the authors' cohort, more than 13.5% of patients who had symptomatic sleep apnea had a diagnosis of heart failure. This finding was in contrast to the parent population, in which only 4.4% were diagnosed as having heart failure. Published epidemiologic studies report associations between OSA and heart failure. Furthermore, the Sleep Health Heart Study showed that subjects who had OSA and an AHI of 11 or more events per hour of sleep were more

Table 1: Comorbid conditions in patients diagnosed as having sleep apnea and in the parent population

	Obstructive sleep apnea	Rest of VHA Beneficiaries (%)	Odds Ratio[a] (95% Confidence Interval)	χ^2 P-value
Comorbid condition	98,735	3,548,593		
Hypertension	59,362 (60.1%)	1,391,965 (39.2%)	2.34 (2.31–2.37)	< .0001
Obesity	30,082 (30.5%)	239,460 (6.8%)	6.06 (5.97–6.14)	< .0001
Diabetes	32,448 (32.9%)	577,512 (16.3%)	2.52 (2.48–2.55)	< .0001
Heart failure	13,281 (13.5%)	151,155 (4.4%)	3.40 (3.34–3.46)	< .0001
Cardiovascular disease	27,247 (27.6%)	596,358 (16.8%)	1.84 (1.82–1.87)	< .0001
Cerebrovascular accident	5631 (5.7%)	132,039 (3.7%)	1.57 (1.52–1.61)	< .0001

[a] Odds ratio adjusted for age, gender, and ethnicity.

likely to have heart failure, independent of other known risk factors [31–33]. Another systemic vascular comorbid condition, diagnosed cerebrovascular accident, also was more prevalent in patients who had sleep apnea than in the parent population. The association between cerebrovascular accident and OSA is well documented in other published literature [31,34–36]. In a recent report on data from the Wisconsin Sleep Cohort Study, high odds ratios for stroke with sleep apnea were found in both cross-sectional and prospective analyses [37].

Summary

Diagnosed sleep apnea is common (2.9%) among VHA beneficiaries. The projected actuarial prevalence may be 16% or more when extrapolated from published data [14]. Further studies are needed to establish the true prevalence of sleep apnea in this population. Accurate information is required for appropriate resource allocation to meet health care needs of VHA beneficiaries. Importantly, strong associations between cardiovascular and other conditions and diagnosed sleep apnea were found, extending previously reported findings to the VHA beneficiary population. While the causal role of sleep apnea in these conditions cannot be determined from these data, our findings stress the need for further studies. Understanding the impact of increased case-finding and therapeutic interventions for sleep apnea on patient outcomes, health care utilization, and cost in this high-risk population remains a high priority.

References

[1] Young T, Palta M, Dempse J, et al. The occurrence of sleep-disordered breathing among middle-aged adults. N Engl J Med 1993;328(17):1230–5.

[2] Guilleminault C, Partinen M, Querasalva MA, et al. Determinants of daytime sleepiness in obstructive sleep-apnea. Chest 1988;94(1):32–7.

[3] Flemons WW, Tsai W. Quality of life consequences of sleep-disordered breathing. J Allergy Clin Immunol 1997;99(2):S750–6.

[4] Findley LJ, Weiss JW, Jabour ER. Drivers with untreated sleep apnea. A cause of death and serious injury. Arch Intern Med 1991;151(7):1451–2.

[5] Quan SF, Howard BV, Iber C, et al. The Sleep Heart Health Study: design, rationale, and methods. Sleep 1997;20(12):1077–85.

[6] Nieto FJ, Young TB, Lind BK, et al. Association of sleep-disordered breathing, sleep apnea, and hypertension in a large community-based study. Sleep Heart Health Study. JAMA 2000;283(14): 1829–36.

[7] Decary A, Rouleau I, Montplaisir J. Cognitive deficits associated with sleep apnea syndrome: a proposed neuropsychological test battery. Sleep 2000;23(3):369–81.

[8] Weaver TE, Laizner AM, Evans LK, et al. An instrument to measure functional status outcomes for disorders of excessive sleepiness. Sleep 1997; 20(10):835–43.

[9] Young T, Peppard PE, Gottlieb DJ. Epidemiology of obstructive sleep apnea: a population health perspective. Am J Respir Crit Care Med 2002; 165(9):1217–39.

[10] Ancoli-Israel S, Kripke DF. Prevalent sleep problems in the aged. Biofeedback Self Regul 1991; 16(4):349–59.

[11] Kreis P, Kripke DF, Ancoli-Israel S. Sleep apnea: a prospective study. West J Med 1983;139(2): 171–3.

[12] Ancoli-Israel S, Kripke DF, Menn SJ, et al. Benefits of a sleep disorders clinic in a Veterans Administration Medical Center. West J Med 1981; 135(1):14–8.

[13] Ashton CM, Souchek J, Petersen NJ, et al. Hospital use and survival among Veterans Affairs beneficiaries. N Engl J Med 2003;349(17): 1637–46.

[14] Sharafkhaneh A, Richardson P, Hirshkowitz M. Sleep apnea in a high risk population: a study of veterans health administration beneficiaries. Sleep Medicine 2004;5(4):345–50.

[15] Young T, Evans L, Finn L, et al. Estimation of the clinically diagnosed proportion of sleep apnea syndrome in middle-aged men and women. Sleep 1997;20(9):705–6.

[16] Bixler EO, Vgontzas AN, Ten Have T, et al. Effects of age on sleep apnea in men. I. Prevalence and severity. Am J Respir Crit Care Med 1998;157(1): 144–8.

[17] Duran J, Esnaola S, Rubio R, et al. Obstructive sleep apnea-hypopnea and related clinical features in a population-based sample of subjects aged 30 to 70 yr. Am J Respir Crit Care Med 2001;163(3 Pt 1):685–9.

[18] Redline S, Young T. Epidemiology and natural history of obstructive sleep apnea. Ear Nose Throat J 1993;72(1):20–6.

[19] Ancoli-Israel S, Kripke DF, Klauber MR, et al. Sleep-disordered breathing in community-dwelling elderly. Sleep 1991;14(6):486–95.

[20] Young T. Sleep-disordered breathing in older adults: is it a condition distinct from that in middle-aged adults? Sleep 1996;19(7):529–30.

[21] Young T, Shahar E, Nieto FJ, et al. Predictors of sleep-disordered breathing in community-dwelling adults: the sleep heart health study. Arch Intern 2002;162(8):893–900.

[22] Strobel RJ, Rosen RC. Obesity and weight loss in obstructive sleep apnea: a critical review. Sleep 1996;19(2):104–15.

[23] Shinohara E, Kihara S, Yamashita S, et al. Visceral fat accumulation as an important risk factor for obstructive sleep apnoea syndrome

in obese subjects. J Intern Med 1997;241(1): 11–8.

[24] Newman AB, Nieto FJ, Guidry U, et al. Relation of sleep-disordered breathing to cardiovascular disease risk factors: the sleep heart health study. Am J Epidemiol 2001;154(1):50–9.

[25] Levinson PD, McGarvey ST, Carlisle CC, et al. Adiposity and cardiovascular risk factors in men with obstructive sleep apnea. Chest 1993; 103(5):1336–42.

[26] Meigs JB. Epidemiology of the metabolic syndrome, 2002. Am J Manag Care 2002;8(11 Suppl):S283–92.

[27] Bixler EO, Vgontzas AN, Lin HM, et al. Association of hypertension and sleep-disordered breathing. Arch Intern Med 2000;160(15): 2289–95.

[28] Young T, Peppard P, Palta M, et al. Population-based study of sleep-disordered breathing as a risk factor for hypertension. Arch Intern Med 1997;157(15):1746–52.

[29] Millman RP, Redline S, Carlisle CC, et al. Daytime hypertension in obstructive sleep apnea. Prevalence and contributing risk factors. Chest 1991;99(4):861–6.

[30] Peppard PE, Young T, Palta M, et al. Prospective study of the association between sleep-disordered breathing and hypertension. N Engl J Med 2000;342(19):1378–84.

[31] Shahar E, Whitney CW, Redline S, et al. Sleep-disordered breathing and cardiovascular disease: cross-sectional results of the Sleep Heart Health Study. Am J Respir Crit Care Med 2001;163(1): 19–25.

[32] Sin DD, Fitzgerald F, Parker JD, et al. Risk factors for central and obstructive sleep apnea in 450 men and women with congestive heart failure. Am J Respir Crit Care Med 1999;160(4):1101–6.

[33] Javaheri S, Parker TJ, Liming JD, et al. Sleep apnea in 81 ambulatory male patients with stable heart failure. Types and their prevalences, consequences, and presentations. Circulation 6–2 1998;97(21):2154–9.

[34] Palomaki H. Snoring and the risk of ischemic brain infarction. Stroke 1991;22(8):1021–5.

[35] Partinen M, Palomaki H. Snoring and cerebral infarction. Lancet 1985;2(8468):1325–6.

[36] Neau JP, Meurice JC, Paquereau J, et al. Habitual snoring as a risk factor for brain infarction. Acta Neurol Scand 1995;92(1):63–8.

[37] Arzt M, Young T, Finn L, et al. Association of sleep-disordered breathing and the occurrence of stroke. Am J Respir Crit Care Med 2005; 172(11):1447–51.

ELSEVIER
SAUNDERS

SLEEP
MEDICINE
CLINICS

Sleep Med Clin 1 (2006) 449–460

Clinical and Laboratory Assessment of Sleep-Related Breathing Disorders

Max Hirshkowitz, PhD, D ABSM[a,b,*],
Amir Sharafkhaneh, MD, D ABSM[a,b], Meir Kryger, MD[c]

- Clinical assessment
  - *Interview*
  - *Questionnaires*
- Laboratory assessment—
  polysomnography

- *Recording*
- *Scoring*
- *Interpretation*
- References

Clinical assessment

Interview

Clinical assessment of a patient who has sleep-related breathing disorders (SRBD) begins with a comprehensive interview. This clinical interview will help identify signs and symptoms as well as establish the patient's routine sleep–wake schedule. The interview also helps the provider make a proper differential diagnosis and prompts ordering relevant diagnostic tests. Furthermore, symptom severity and signs of daytime impairment will guide cautionary recommendations about the hazards of sleepiness, sleeplessness, and sleep-related behaviors.

Sleep schedule

Determining the underlying etiology in a patient complaining of sleepiness, sleeplessness, or sleep-related behaviors begins with information about the individual's sleep schedule. A good place to start is learning what time they retire to sleep and what time they awaken on weekdays (or workdays). This should be compared with begin and end times for the sleep period on weekends to determine if the individual is extending or shortening their sleep schedule duration, phase advancing or delaying their schedule, or both. A pattern of sleep fasting during the week and binging on weekends is common in our sleep-deprived society. Sometimes sleepiness will seem far out of proportion to the level of pathophysiology revealed by polysomnography; however, knowing the sleep schedule can elucidate the matter. Finally, the clinician should find out how often the patient naps and for how long. It is helpful to know if the naps are refreshing or unrefreshing.

Sleep problems

The mnemonic device "BEARS" has been suggested as an interview guide for trainees. The B stands for bedtime, the E for excessive sleepiness, the A for

---

[a] Baylor College of Medicine, 1 Baylor Plaza, Houston, TX 77030, USA
[b] Sleep Disorders & Research Center, Michael E. DeBakey Veterans Affairs Medical Center (111i), 2002 Holcombe Blvd., Houston, TX 77030, USA
[c] Saint Boniface General Hospital Sleep Laboratory & University of Manitoba, Winnipeg, Canada
* Corresponding author. Sleep Center (111i), 2002 Holcombe Blvd., Bldg. 100, Rm 6C344, Houston, TX 77030.
E-mail address: maxh@bcm.tmc.edu (M. Hirshkowitz).

1556-407X/06/$ – see front matter © 2006 Elsevier Inc. All rights reserved.
sleep.theclinics.com

doi:10.1016/j.jsmc.2006.11.005

night and early morning awakenings, the R for regularity and duration of sleep, and the S for snoring. Critical information for recognizing sleep apnea include: (1) loud disruptive snoring with frequent nocturnal awakenings, (2) awakening at night with choking or gasping, (3) witnessed apnea (bed partner, friends, family members), (4) excessive daytime sleepiness, and (5) a history of falling asleep when driving or when at stop lights.

Overall, there are many sleep disorders, often with overlapping symptoms. A thorough sleep history is essential. The authors routinely ask patients to complete a sleep questionnaire before the interview. The completed questionnaire guides the interview whereby more detailed follow-up questions are asked for sleep problems that were affirmed. Table 1 shows signs and symptoms one should address when obtaining a sleep history.

Medical and family history

Risk factors for sleep-related breathing disorders include being middle-aged or older, being male, being overweight, having micro- or retrognathia, a large tongue, a low set soft palate, or a crowded airway. Postmenopausal women not taking hormone replacement therapy may be at risk and often complain of insomnia rather than sleepiness. Sleep-related breathing disorders are commonly associated with hypertension, heart disease, lung disease, diabetes, neurologic, metabolic, and psychiatric conditions. Some sleep disorders are familial or genetic; therefore, having a good medical and family history is essential.

Medications

The clinician should conduct a complete medication inventory on the patient. Medications with soporific properties should particularly be noted. Similarly, stimulant and other wake-promoting medication use must be considered (Table 2).

Questionnaires

Sleep questionnaire

A wide variety of sleep questionnaires exist, and many sleep disorders centers and laboratories develop their own instruments. Figs. 1 and 2 show the authors' sleep center's screening questionnaire and sleep problems checklist. Validated sleep questionnaires include the Sleep Disorders Questionnaire and the Pittsburgh Sleep Questionnaire.

Sleepiness questionnaire

It can be helpful to index sleepiness with a validated instrument. The Epworth Sleepiness Scale is the most widely used questionnaire in clinical practice. However, other choices exist, including the Karolinska Questionnaire, the Stanford Sleepiness Scale,

the Profile of Mood States, the Pictorial Sleepiness Questionnaire, the Berlin Questionnaire, and a variety of digital–analog scales. The authors consider an Epworth score ranging from 8 to 11 (inclusive) as mild sleepiness, from 12 to 15 as moderate sleepiness, and 16 or above as severe sleepiness. These categories are based on a survey of more than 3000 healthy adults and an equal number of patients who have sleep disorders. In cases where the patient is a commercial driver or operates dangerous machinery, one might want to conduct a maintenance of wakefulness test, an objective test of alertness.

The cause of sleepiness is multifactorial. It depends on prior sleep duration, quality, and timing (within the circadian rhythm). Sleep deprivation, sleep disruption, dysfunction in central alertness mechanisms, medication (and recreational drugs including alcohol), diet, and exercise regimen all can contribute to sleepiness.

Depression questionnaire

Sleep-related breathing disorders and mood disorders are commonly associated. Depression and insomnia are comorbid with as much as 90% of patients who have major depressive disorder suffering from sleeplessness. Furthermore, mood disorders may act as a barrier to good adherence with positive airway pressure therapy. It is prudent to administer a depression-screening test as part of a sleep disorders evaluation. Popular screening tools include the Beck Depression Inventory and the Zung Depression Scale.

Laboratory assessment—polysomnography

Attended laboratory polysomnography is currently the standard technique for diagnosing SRBD.

Recording

Sleep stages

Electroencephalograhic (EEG) activity recorded from central (C3 or C4) and occipital (O3 or O4) derivations, electro-oculographic (EOG) activity from right and left eye (recorded from the outer canthi), and submental electromyographic (EMG) are used to define sleep stage. In standard practice, each 30 seconds of recording (1 epoch) is categorized as wakefulness or sleep stage 1, 2, 3, 4, or rapid eye movement (REM). Epoch length was a convention based on paper polygraph tracings. These tracings were usually recorded at a chart speed of 10 mm/s; therefore, each resulting polygraph page was 30 seconds in duration. Because each polygraph page is numbered, it was a matter of convenience to summarize sleep state for each 30-second page. Although paper polysomnograms

Table 1: **Signs and symptoms of sleep disorders**

Question	SRBD	NAR	INSOM	RLS or PLMD	PARA or SEIZ
Snoring	×				
Unrefreshing sleep	×		×	×	×
Witnessed apnea	×				×
Waking up choking or gasping for air	×				
Nocturnal reflux	×				
Nocturia	×				
Nocturnal sweating	×				
Sleep talking	×				×
Morning dry mouth	×				
Morning headache	×				×
Sleep onset insomnia			×		
Sleep maintenance insomnia		×	×		
Early orning awakenings			×		
Rumination at sleep onset			×		
Worrying about things while in bed			×		
Fear of not being able to fall asleep			×		
Fear of not being able to fall back to sleep			×		
Unexpected sleep onset	×	×			
Sleep attacks (sudden irresistible sleep)		×			
Falling asleep while driving	×	×			
Muscle weakness provoked by laughter		×			
Muscle weakness triggered by strong emotion		×			
Waking up with paralysis (unable to move)		×			
Paralysis while falling asleep		×			
Floating images as you are falling asleep		×			
Floating images as you are just waking up		×			
Floating images that persist when eyes are open		×			
Teeth grinding					×
Leg cramps (Charley horse)					×
Crawling sensations in legs when resting				×	
Leg crawling sensation relieved by movement				×	
Leg kicking at night				×	
Nightmares (extremely frightening dreams)					×
Sleep Terror (awaken frightened, no dream)					×
Acting out dream (dream enactment)					×
Dream enactment with arm flailing or leg moving					×
Dream enactment with injury					×
Tongue biting in sleep (bloody pillow)					×
Nocturnal awaking with dystonic posturing					×
Routine napping	×	×			
Unrefreshing naps	×				

Abbreviations: INSOM, insomnia; NAR, narcolepsy; PARA, parasomnia; PLMD, periodic limb movement disorder; RLS, restless legs syndrome; SEIZ, seizure disorder; SRBD, sleep-related breathing disorders.

Table 2: Stimulant and sedating substances

Stimulants and wake-promoting substances	Sedative-hypnotics and other sleep-promoting substances
Methylphenidate	Zaleplon
Modafinil	Zolpedim
Amphetamine	Zopiclone
Methamphetamines	Eszopiclone
Dextroamphetamine	Halcion
Levoamphetamine	Temazepam
Selegiline	Estazolam
Mazindol	Quazepam
Pemoline	Flurazepam
Caffeine	Chloral Hydrate
Theobromine	Alcohol
Many of the SSRIs	Diphenhydramine
	Trazodone
	Amitriptyline
	Doxepin
	Mirtazipine
	Quitiapine
	Most BZDs
	Most TCAs
	Most Neuroleptics

Abbreviations: BZD, benzodiazepine; SSRI, selective serotonin reuptake inhibitor; TCA, tricyclic antidepressant.

have mostly gone the way of the dinosaurs, the practice of 30-second epoch sleep staging continues, notwithstanding computerized polygraph systems' ability to easily resize pages and alter temporal resolution.

Airflow

Pneumotachography The pneumotachograph can provide quantitative measures of airflow. Several types of pneumotachographs exist; however, the most common type uses differential pressure airflow transducers. Airflow is directed through a cylinder. Before exiting the cylinder, air passes through a small resistive field, usually small parallel tubes or a grill that promotes laminar flow. A differential manometer measures the pressure drop across this resistive field. The pneumotachograph is usually connected to a facemask. Although this pneumotachograph and facemask combination is the most accurate means of assessing the volume of airflow, it is a relatively large uncomfortable device, making it generally unsuitable for routine sleep evaluations. Some positive airway pressure machines have built-in pneumotachographs and can be used to monitor airflow (albeit uncalibrated) and cardiogenic oscillations (a central apnea feature).

Nasal airway pressure Compared with atmospheric pressure, airway pressure is negative during inspiration and positive during expiratory. Many laboratories use nasal pressure changes as a surrogate measure of airflow. Nasal pressure also seems more sensitive to flow limitation than thermistors. Flow limitation is inferred when the signal plateaus during inspiration. Some patients, however, do not breathe through their nose; therefore, additional instrumentation is needed to assess flow.

Thermistors and thermocouples Under normal circumstances, the air inside the body is warmer than the air outside the body (unless one is in south Texas during the summer and the air conditioning is broken). The body's core temperature passively heats the air in the lungs. Thermistors can be used to detect exhalation of this warm air at the nares and mouth and inhalation of cooler (ambient temperature) air. A thermistor is a thermally sensitive resistor whereby increased resistance from warming can be transduced to voltage and displayed polygraphically.

Expired carbon dioxide sensing Air leaving the lungs has a much higher concentration of CO_2 than ambient air. There is always a large CO_2 difference between air entering versus exiting the respiratory system. Consequently, expiration can be estimated by measuring CO_2 in front of the nose and mouth. The pressure offers several advantages over measuring nasal pressure or using thermistors. First, the end of breath concentration may yield an end-tidal P_{CO_2}. Because the catheters sampling CO_2 may also entrain room air, the measured is likely to be lower than the end-tidal P_{CO_2}. Thus, an elevated P_{CO_2} should be accepted as real, indicating that true P_{CO_2} is even higher. This is the only noninvasive measurement sampling the airstream that can potentially confirm hypoventilation. Second, the shape of the expired curve may offer useful information. When a patient originally demonstrates an expired CO_2 curve with a clearcut plateau, the loss of the plateau or the curve becoming smaller or dome-shaped indicates a change in breathing pattern, usually a reduction in expiratory volume. Third, during central apnea, the CO_2 tracing may show cardiogenic oscillations. These oscillations are the result of small-volume displacements caused by the beating heart. These oscillations are synchronized to the heartbeat, and they prove that the upper airway is wide open. The catheter system should be of low volume and the analyzer set on its fastest response to detect these oscillations.

Respiratory effort

Rib cage and abdominal motion During normal breathing, inspiratory diaphragm muscles contract causing rib cage expansion and downward movement of the diaphragm. These movements produce a negative intrathoracic pressure that causes airflow

Sleep Center Screening Questionnaire(v601)

Patient Name _____   Date _____

EPWORTH SLEEPINESS SCALE

How LIKELY are you to DOZE off or FALL ASLEEP in the following situations, in contrast to feeling just tired? This refers to your usual way of life in recent times. Even if you have not done some of these things recently, try to work out how they would have affected you. Please check one box per line.

--- CHANCE OF DOZING OFF ---

Never	Slight	Moderate	High	
☐	☐	☐	☐	Sitting and reading
☐	☐	☐	☐	Watching TV
☐	☐	☐	☐	Sitting, inactive in a public place (example, a theater or a meeting)
☐	☐	☐	☐	As a passenger in a car for an hour without a break
☐	☐	☐	☐	Lying down to rest in the afternoon when circumstances permit
☐	☐	☐	☐	Sitting and talking to someone
☐	☐	☐	☐	Sitting quietly after lunch without alcohol
☐	☐	☐	☐	In a car, while stopped for a few minutes in traffic

BRIEF SLEEP SYMPTOM CHECKLIST *(Please check the boxes that best describes you)*

Never	Rarely	Frequently	Always	
☐	☐	☐	☐	I snore loudly
☐	☐	☐	☐	I awaken gasping or choking for breath
☐	☐	☐	☐	I awaken in the morning unrefreshed
☐	☐	☐	☐	I have problems falling asleep or staying asleep (insomnia)
☐	☐	☐	☐	My sleep is very restless
☐	☐	☐	☐	My sleep is distrubed by unusual behaviors (for example: nightmares, sleepwalking, dream enactments, tongue biting, bedwetting... etc.)
☐	☐	☐	☐	I fall asleep while driving
☐	☐	☐	☐	I've been told that I stop breathing in my sleep (told by _____)

SLEEP SCHEDULE *(Please provide the following information)*

What time do you go to bed on WEEKDAYS? _____ AM or PM   Do you nap? **[Yes] [No]**

What time do you get up on WEEKDAYS? _____ AM or PM   How often do you nap? _____ times per week

What time do you go to bed on WEEKENDS? _____ AM or PM   How long are the naps? _____ minutes

What time do you get up on WEEKENDS? _____ AM or PM   Do you awaken refreshed? **[Yes] [No]**

Are you a shift worker? **[Yes] [No]** If yes, what kind of shift do you work?_____

Developed by Max Hirshkowitz @ Flatland Logic Group

Fig. 1. Sleep center screening questionnaire. (Courtesy of Max Hirshkowitz, PhD, Houston, TX.)

into the lung. Thus, a change in lung volume is the sum of the volume changes of the structures surrounding the lungs, the rib cage, and the abdomen. Some mistakenly interpret the abdominal and rib cage motion changes to imply separate activity of abdominal and thoracic respiratory muscles; however, this is not the case. Most changes in abdominal and rib cage volumes (including paradoxical motion) can be explained by changes in the respiratory muscles directly inserting onto the thoracic cage.

During normal unobstructed breathing, the enlargement of the thorax and the outward movement of the abdominal wall occur together (ie, they are *in phase*). If calibrated, one can quantify the change in rib cage and abdominal volume and determine the relative contributions of the rib cage and abdominal compartments. Assuming constancy for

Sleep Problems Checklist (v0406)

Patient Name _____   Date _____

What problem causes you to seek our help and how does it affect your life? _____
_____
_____

CHECK the box for each problem you CURRENTLY HAVE.

☐ Loud snoring with frequent awakenings
☐ Crawling feelings in legs when trying to sleep
☐ Leg-kicking during sleep
☐ Leg cramps in sleep
☐ Trouble falling asleep at night
☐ Trouble staying asleep at night
☐ Racing thoughts when trying to sleep
☐ Increased muscle tension when trying to sleep
☐ Fear of being unable to sleep
☐ Laying in bed worrying when trying to sleep
☐ Waking too early in the morning
☐ Sleep talking
☐ Sweating a lot at night
☐ Waking up with reflux (and/or heartburn)
☐ Waking up to urinate 2 or more times nightly
☐ Nightmares

☐ Teethgrinding during sleep
☐ Morning headaches
☐ Morning dry mouth
☐ Sleepwalking
☐ Tongue biting in sleep
☐ Bedwetting
☐ Acting out dreams
☐ Uncontrollable daytime sleep attacks
☐ Falling asleep unexpectedly
☐ Falling asleep at work
☐ Falling asleep at school
☐ I use sleeping pills to help me sleep
☐ I use alcohol to help me sleep
☐ Pain interfering with sleep
    where is the pain?
    _____

For each symptom, please CHECK the boxes that BEST DESCRIBES YOU

Never	Rarely	Sometimes	Usually	Always	
☐	☐	☐	☐	☐	When falling asleep, I feel paralyzed (unable to move)
☐	☐	☐	☐	☐	I feel unable to move (paralyzed) after a nap
☐	☐	☐	☐	☐	I have dream-like images (hallucinations) when I awaken in the morning even though I know I am not asleep
☐	☐	☐	☐	☐	I see vivid dream-like (hallucinations) either just before or just after a daytime nap, yet I am sure I am awake when they happen
☐	☐	☐	☐	☐	I am often unable to move (paralyzed) when I am waking up in the morning
☐	☐	☐	☐	☐	I get "weak knees" when I laugh
☐	☐	☐	☐	☐	I get sudden muscular weakness (or even brief periods of paralysis, being unable to move) when laughing, angry, or in situations of strong emotion

Developed by Max Hirshkowitz @ Flatland Logic Group

Fig. 2. Sleep problems checklist. (Courtesy of Max Hirshkowitz, PhD, Houston, TX.)

abdominal and rib cage fractional contributions, quantitative calculation of air exchange is possible. However, postural and muscle changes compromise accuracy because calibration will change during the night.

Pleural pressure Some laboratories use esophageal pressure to measure inspiratory effort. Many patients do not tolerate this procedure. However, newer, thin, catheter-tip piezoelectric transducers appear to be tolerated. Measuring esophageal pressure during inspiration can provide the sensitive measures needed to diagnosis of the upper airway resistance syndrome. The classic findings show pleural pressure becoming progressively negative until an arousal occurs (sometimes associated with an audible snort). Postarousal pleural pressure swings decrease, but soon the cycle of increasing pressure swings leading up to arousal starts again.

Respiratory muscle electromyography Electromyography recordings from the chest wall can be used to index respiratory effort. Electrode pairs are placed in an intercostal space on the right anterior chest until an optimal signal is attained; this may require trial and error.

Lung volume

There are various techniques with which lung volume can be estimated or measured. These techniques employ strain gauges, inductance plethysmography, impedance pneumography, static charge sensitive beds, magnetometers, body plethysmographs, and barometric methods. Calibration procedures can be involved and time consuming but yield quantitative data. Consequently, lung volume measurement methods are mainly the province of research centers. The transducer (eg, strain gauges and inductance plethysmography bands), however, are not strangers to clinically oriented sleep centers, but they are mostly to record rib cage movement to detect respiratory effort.

Oxygenation

Indwelling arterial catheter Measuring oxygen content directly from blood sampled from an indwelling arterial catheter during sleep is invasive and impractical for routine use at clinical sleep laboratories. Furthermore, sampling would not be adequate to detect the transient changes occurring in response to sleep-related respiratory events.

Pulse oximetry Noninvasive technologies allow the continuous monitoring of oxygen saturation of arterial blood (Sao_2). Pulse oximetry represents standard technique for recording oxyhemoglobin desaturations during polysomnography. Pulse oximeters determine Sao_2 using spectrophotoelectrical techniques by way of 2-wavelength light transmitter and receiver placed on either side of a pulsating arterial vascular bed. Manufacturers recommend digit, ear, and nasal sites. The amplitude of light detected by the receiver is dependent on the magnitude of the change in arterial pulse, the wavelengths transmitted through the arterial vascular bed, and the Sao_2 of the arterial hemoglobin. These devices are sensitive only to tissues that pulsate; thus, venous blood, connective tissue, skin pigment, and bone theoretically do not interfere with Sao_2 measurement. A minimal pulse amplitude must be detected by the devices to prevent erroneous measurements. Dyshemoglobinemias, however, may

cause problems. The correct alignment of the light transmitter and receiver is critical to the proper operation of pulse oximeters. If the sensor is applied to a digit, that digit must be immobilized. Significant bending of the digit may restrict the ability of the devices to detect pulsatile flow, the absence of which precludes Sao_2 determinations. Although all pulse oximeters are based on similar technology, they have very different response characteristics.

In reflectance pulse oximetry, the light transmitter and receiver are on the same surface. The light transmitted into the vascular bed is scattered, absorbed, and reflected. Thus only a small proportion of the light returns to the receiver. Reflectance devices deal with weaker pulse signals and therefore are more sensitive to changes in blood pressure and motion artifacts.

For most adults, the ear is the preferred location. Recording from the ear also helps to reduce circulator delay. This becomes especially important for associating the respiratory and desaturation event when apnea episodes occur in rapid succession, or the patient has congestive heart failure.

Most pulse oximeters filter the Sao_2 signal. For some devices, the filter algorithms use the heart rate; thus, the degree of filtering becomes inversely related to rate, and at very low heart rates, the signal is heavily filtered. The greater the filtering, the less likely is the detection of brief, mild hypoxemic episodes. The least filtering (ie, the fastest response or the highest sampling rate) should be used so that transient changes are not missed.

Because pulse oximeters use 2 wavelengths of light in the process of estimating Sao_2, they are unable to distinguish three or more hemoglobin species. In the presence of carboxyhemoglobin, the Sao_2 will be overestimated in heavy smokers, whose carboxyhemoglobin level may reach 10% to 20%. In the presence of a rising methemoglobin concentration, Sao_2 measured by oximetry will plateau toward 85%, regardless of whether the true Sao_2 is much higher or lower. Because light is transmitted through tissue, pigment in the skin may degrade oximeter performance with the device indicating a "probe off" or "perfusion low" message. Although probe connectors from one manufacturer may perfectly fit into the unit of another, the wiring may be incompatible, and severe burns may result. Pressure-related injuries to the digits have also been reported.

Transcutaneous oxygen and carbon dioxide The estimation of Pao_2 from the surface of the skin is dependent on the oxygen flux through the skin, local oxygen consumption, and the diffusion barrier of the skin. This measurement technique is most commonly used in neonates, whose skin is thin.

The accuracy of transcutaneous measurement also depends on correct sensor application. To precisely convert $tcPO_2$ measurements to PaO_2 values, a calibration curve for each subject is required; this is a prohibitive step. In practice, the $tcPO_2$ measurements are thus used to track, in relative terms, the status of arterial oxygen content. The responsiveness of the device is not adequate to rapidly track the blood gas changes of short apneas (less than 30 seconds) because oxygen diffuses slowly across the skin. The conditions that govern the transcutaneous measurement of PCO_2 are similar to those described for PaO_2. Transcutaneous blood gas determinations are of greatest value in neonates. The use of transcutaneous PCO_2 is to assess hypoventilation and its treatment in adults and children.

Cardiac rhythm

Cardiac rhythm is usually monitored with a single modified precordial lead. The purpose is principally recorded as a safety measure. Significant electrocardiographic abnormalities should be noted in the patient's chart and polysomnographic report. Potentially fatal arrhythmias may prompt referral for further workup if the patient is not already in the care of a specialist. Asystoles, Vtach, Afib, and a variety of blocks are not uncommon in patients who have severe sleep-related breathing disorders (Fig. 3).

Leg movements

Leg movement activity should be recorded according to standard technique [1]. Leg movement recordings are usually made using two surface electrodes placed on each leg. Electrodes are positioned on the anterior tibialis muscle 2 to 4 cm apart to detect flexion of the great toe, ankle, knee, or hip. Electrode impedance should be between 10,000 and 30,000 ohms, time constant should be set to 0.003, low frequency filter between 5 and 10 Hz, high frequency filter above 100 Hz, and sensitivity approximately 50 μV/cm. Recordings from both the left and right legs should be made because leg movements can occur on one leg and may not be present on the other. The recordings from the left and right legs can be kept on separate channels or can be combined onto a single tracing. The leg movement recordings are made to determine if the patient has comorbid periodic limb movement disorder. In some cases, the leg movement disorder resolves after the sleep-related breathing disorder is well treated. Patients who have periodic limb movement disorder often complain of restless and nonrefreshing sleep. If the leg movement disorder persists, it may undermine treatment efforts for the sleep-related breathing disorder.

Scoring

Staging

Sleep stages should be scored according to standardized technique [2]. *Wakefulness* (ie, stage W or stage 0) with eyes closed is accompanied by an electroencephalograph rhythm predominantly in the alpha range. Some individuals do not have distinct alpha activity and transition quickly to a low-voltage mixed-frequency activity. *Sleep onset epoch* is determined when alpha duration decreases to less than 50% of an epoch or a vertex wave, K-complex, sleep spindle, or delta activity occurs, otherwise, wakefulness is scored. *Stage 1 sleep* is scored when low-voltage mixed-frequency EEG is present but there are no K-complexes, spindles, or REMs. Stage 1 sleep is a nonalpha state with EEG activity that is deltaless and spindleless; however, vertex sharp waves may be present. *Stage 2 sleep* epochs are classified when there are sleep spindles or K-complexes but high-amplitude (75 μV or greater) delta EEG activity occupies less than 20% of the epoch. *Stage 3* is designated when there is 20% to 50% delta (or slow wave activity) in an epoch. *Stage 4* is scored when

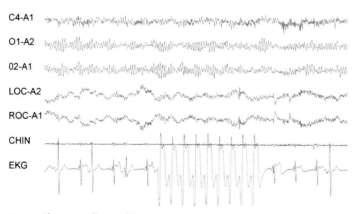

Fig. 3. Electrocardiographic report.

delta activity covers more than 50% of an epoch. REM sleep is scored when eye movements and muscle atonia accompany a stage 1 EEG pattern. Sawtooth theta waves may also accompany REM sleep. In addition to rapid eye movements, other physiologic activities accompany REM sleep, including middle ear muscle activity, periorbital integrated potentials, and sleep-related erections. There are periods within REM sleep when eye movement activity, and presumably other phasic event activity, is high. At other times, REM-like EEG activity continues with very little phasic activity. These two faces of REM sleep are called *phasic REM sleep* and *tonic REM sleep*. Stages 1, 2, 3, and 4 are sometimes collectively referred to as *non-REM* sleep (NREM). Stages 1 and 2 are sometimes referred to as *light sleep,* and stage 3 and 4 are often combined and called *slow wave sleep* or *deep sleep.* Table 3 summarizes EEG-EOG-EMG characteristics for wakefulness and the different sleep stages.

Sleep stage scoring is mainly used to separate wakefulness, REM sleep, and NREM sleep (Fig. 4). In most patients, the severity of obstructive sleep apnea increases during REM sleep. Sometimes REM sleep is suppressed by the breathing disorder. To gauge overall severity, the rate, duration, and concomitant changes associated with the sleep-disordered breathing events must be determined during both REM and NREM sleep. Interestingly, the typical pattern of greater severity during REM sleep is reversed in some patients who have heart disease. In particular, patients who have congestive heart failure will have more normal breathing during REM compared with NREM sleep.

Central nervous system arousals

Central nervous system (CNS) arousals should be scored according to standard technique [3]. Arousal scoring is specific and unambiguous; however "variants" have emerged that rely heavily on EMG or that consider autonomic nervous system activation. Ten seconds of uninterrupted sleep must precede an arousal. A second arousal can be scored only if there is 10 seconds or more of intervening sleep. Scoring criteria require specific presence of a minimum 3-second shift in EEG frequency to score an arousal. When artifact, K-complexes or delta waves are accompanied by a 3-second shift in EEG frequency; these occurrences are also scored as arousals. However, a K-complex or delta burst alone does not constitute an arousal. Although chin EMG amplitude is not used to score an arousal from NREM sleep, increased chin EMG amplitude is often present. Because sleep stage scoring rules specifically state that alpha activity greater than one half the epoch must be scored as stage wake, arousals can terminate in stage wake because the duration criteria is 3 seconds or greater.

Respiratory events

Apnea   Apnea has been clearly defined in the literature for many years as a cessation of nasal/oral airflow for 10 seconds or more [4,5]. Apnea episodes can be classified as obstructive, central, or mixed. An *obstructive apnea* is characterized by complete or near complete cessation of nasal/oral airflow with continued or increased respiratory effort (Fig. 5). The obstruction is caused by narrowing and/or collapse of the upper airway. Asynchronous

Table 3: EEG-EOG-EMG characteristics of sleep and wakefulness

REM Stage	EEG characteristics	EOG	EMG muscle activity
W	Predominant alpha activity (more than 50% of the epoch) mixed with EEG beta	Slow & rapid	High
1	Alpha activity is replaced by low voltage, predominant low voltage, mixed-frequency background activity sometimes with vertex sharp waves	Slow	Decreased from awake
2	Sleep spindles and K-complexes in a background EEG that has less than 20% delta activity	None	Decreased from awake
3	Slow wave (EEG delta activity) comprises 20%–50% of the epoch; sleep spindles usually are present	None	Decreased from awake
4	More than 50% of the epoch has EEG delta activity	None	Decreased from awake
REM	Low voltage, mixed frequency background activity; saw-tooth theta waves may be present	Rapid	Nearly absent

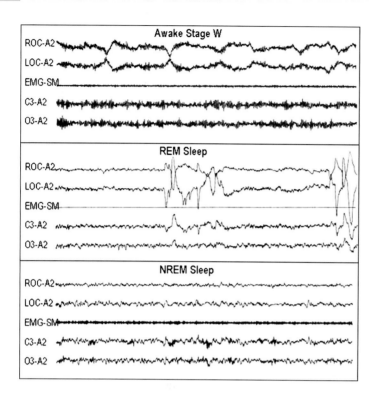

Fig. 4. EEG-EOG-EMG Polysomnographic tracings for wakefulness, REM sleep, and NREM sleep. The figure shows a 30-second tracing of right and left electrooculogram, submentalis electromyogram, and monopolar central and occipital electroencepahlograms (C2–A2 & O3–A2, respectively). ROC, right outer canthus; LOC, left outer canthus; EMG-SM, electromyogram-submentalis.

(paradoxical) breathing may occur during airway obstruction. There may be crescendo snoring leading up to the obstructive event. Obstructive apneas are usually accompanied by oxygen desaturation and terminate with an arousal. A *central apnea* is characterized by complete or near complete cessation of nasal/oral airflow and respiratory effort (Fig. 6). They can result from neurologic

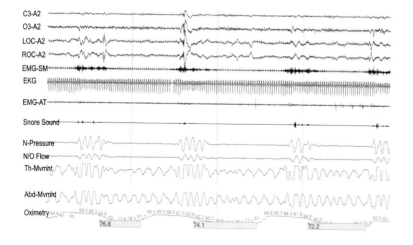

Fig. 5. Obstructive sleep apnea. This 2-minute segment of an overnight sleep study shows a sequence of four consecutive episodes of obstructive sleep apnea. Note the cessation of breathing revealed by nasal pressure (N-Pressure) and nasal/oral airflow (N/O flow) channels notwithstanding continued respiratory effort shown by thoracic movement (Th-Mvmnt) and abdominal movement (Abd-Mvmnt). Blood oxygen saturation (Oximetry) dips as low as 72.2% in response to the third event depicted. Sleep disturbance (arousal) can be observed following each apnea episode and coincident with resumption of breathing on the top five recording channels: central (C2-A2) and occipital (O3-A2) electroencephalogram; left and right eye electro-oculogram (left outer canthus [LOC-A2] and right outer cantus [ROC-A2]); and chin electromyogram (electromyogram-submentalis [EMG-SM]). Snoring sounds (probably from choking, gasping, or an explosive breath) accompany resumption of breathing. Also shown are channels for electrocardiogram (EKG) and leg movements (electromyogram-anterior tibialis [EMG-AT]).

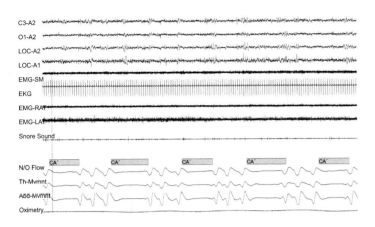

C3-A2
O1-A2
LOC-A2
LOC-A1
EMG-SM
EKG
EMG-RAT
EMG-LAT
Snore Sound

N/O Flow
Th-Mvmnt
Abd-Mvmnt
Oximetry

Fig. 6. Central sleep apnea. This 2-minute segment of an overnight sleep study shows a sequence of five consecutive episodes of central sleep apnea. Note the cessation of breathing revealed by nasal/oral airflow (N/O flow) channels coincident with pauses in respiratory effort shown by thoracic movement (Th-Mvmnt) and abdominal movement (Abd-Mvmnt). Blood oxygen saturation (Oximetry) fluctuates only slightly in response to the apnea episodes. In contrast to obstructive events, these central apnea episodes do not routinely terminate with a sleep disturbance (arousal), as can be seen on the top five recording channels: central (C2-A2) and occipital (O3-A2) electroencephalogram; left and right eye electro-oculogram (left outer canthus [LOC-A2] and right outer cantus [ROC-A2]); and chin electromyogram (electromyogram-submentalis [EMG-SM]). No resumption of breathing-related snoring sounds are noted. Also shown are channels for electrocardiogram (EKG) and right and left leg movements (electromyogram-right anterior tibialis [EMG-RAT] and electromyogram-left anterior tibialis [EMG-LAT]).

dysfunction, medullary pH receptor damage, heart failure, metabolic disorders, of decreased respiratory drive set-point at sleep onset. Oxygen desaturation or arousal may not be associated with the event. A *mixed apnea* contains features of both central and obstructive apnea. Usually beginning as a central apnea, it evolves into an obstructive event. A mixed apnea should lack respiratory effort for at least 25% of its duration.

Hypopnea   In the most general terms, a hypopnea is a shallow breath representing decreased tidal volume. Like apnea, hypopneas can be central or obstructive; however, most of the time they result from partial airway occlusion or increased airway resistance. If a hypopnea is associated with either a disturbance of sleep (arousal, ascending stage shift, or awakening) or a significant oxyhemoglobin desaturation, it is considered pathophysiologic.

As straightforward and logical as this may seem, the specifics of the definition for hypopnea have become controversial. The problem arises from recording technique (ie, using thermistors and thermocouples to assess airflow). These uncalibrated devices do not provide signals that are linear (or even proportional) with tidal volume. Guilleminault's [4] originally defined hypopnea as a reduction in airflow without complete cessation of breathing. This left the question open of how much airflow decrease is needed to score a hypopnea. Similarly, Gould and colleagues [6] described hypopnea as a partial airway obstruction leading to a reduction in tidal volume. Subsequent definitions for hypopnea stipulated a 30% decrease from

baseline in the polygraphic amplitude whereas others required a 50% decrease. In reality, the amplitude cut-point for defining hypopnea is arbitrary, and different laboratories adopted different amplitude criteria for their operational definition. Consequently, it was more shocking than surprising when Moser and colleagues's survey found that no two sleep laboratories used the same definition for hypopnea [7]. Nonetheless, although definitions differ, sleep specialists generally agreed that a hypopnea producing and arousal or oxygen desaturation was bad for sleep.

Then in 2001, the American Academy of Sleep Medicine Clinical Practice Review Committee published a definition for hypopnea largely drawn from Sleep Heart Health epidemiologic studies [8]. This definition was subsequently adopted by Medicare and proclaimed hypopnea as having a 30% reduction from baseline in thoracoabdominal effort or airflow lasting 10 seconds or more and being accompanied by a 4% or greater oxygen desaturation. This definition was a radical departure from previous scoring practice in its requirement of desaturation and complete disregard for sleep disturbance by arousal.

Respiratory effort–related arousals   The 2001 redefinition of hypopnea and its acceptance by Medicare had far-reaching effects. It created an immediate need to create a term that would count those respiratory events previously known as hypopnea but that no longer qualified as such because they lacked a 4% drop in oxygen saturation. Thought leaders immediately seized on the unwieldy appellation "respiratory effort–related arousal," which had been previously created by the Chicago Group as part of their research guidelines for recording and scoring sleep-disordered breathing. Respiratory effort-related arousal is a breathing event in which esophageal pressure becomes increasingly negative for 10 seconds or longer, terminating with a change to less negative pressure with coincident arousal [9]. Clinicians often identify respiratory effort-related arousals using paradoxical breathing as a surrogate measure for increasing negative esophageal pressure. Nasal pressure monitoring provides another noninvasive technique for detecting increased upper airway resistance with increasing negative pressure [10]. Some data indicate that the nasal cannula pressure transducer is as accurate in detecting respiratory effort-related arousals as esophageal manometry [11].

Snoring   Snoring is the sound produced by vibration of the palate and other soft tissues in the oropharynx [12] and usually indicates increased airway resistance. Snoring microphones or snoring vibration sensors can detect snoring during sleep. Snoring without arousals is of unknown clinical consequences; however, arousals associated with snoring are potentially important sleep-disordered breathing events. Thus, it is important to note the presence of snoring and to determine the snore arousal index (number of events associated with arousal per hour of total sleep time).

Interpretation

Interpreting a sleep evaluation involves reviewing the polysomnogram page by page, noting any significant cardiac arrhythmias, determining if there is any epileptiform activity, and checking for evidence of a comorbid movement disorder. Several parameters are calculated to index the level of sleep-disordered breathing activity. The first is apnea index. Apnea index is the number of apnea episodes per hour of sleep. Apnea + hypopnea index is the number of apnea and hypopnea episodes per hour of sleep. Oxygen Desatration Index represents the number of oxyhemoglobin desaturation events per hour of sleep. However, perhaps the most important index is the overall Respiratory Disturbance Index, which is the number of apnea + hypopnea + respiratory effort-related arousals per hour of sleep. It is also helpful to know the minimum SaO_2, the amount of time spent with oxygen level below 85%, and the snore arousal index.

The respiratory disturbance index and other indices during REM sleep versus NREM sleep should be considered. Also, respiratory disturbance index and other indices while sleeping supine can be helpful to determine worse case severity, especially the respiratory disturbance index while supine during REM sleep (if the two occurred concomitantly). The frequency and type of cardiac abnormalities and the depth of desaturation are critical parameters. Finally, correlating the laboratory findings with interview and questionnaire data complete the interpretation. The presence of sleepiness (Epworth Sleepiness Scale score), the number of desaturation events below 88%, 85%, or 80%, and presence of comorbid conditions (eg, hypertension, heart disease, lung disease, depression, or diabetes) figure into selection and aggressiveness of treatment.

References

[1] Sleep Disorders Atlas Task Force. Recording and scoring leg movements. Sleep 1993;16(3): 748–59.

[2] Rechtscaffen A, Kales A. A manual of standardized terminology, techniques and scoring system for sleep stages of human subjects. Los Angeles (CA): Brain Information Service; 1968.

[3] Arousal Scoring Rules Sleep Disorders Atlas Task Force. EEG arousals. Scoring rules and examples—a preliminary report from the Sleep Disorders Atlas Task Force of the American Sleep Disorders Association. Sleep 1992;15(2): 173–84.

[4] Guilleminault C. Sleeping and waking disorders: indications and techniques. Menlo Park (CA): Addison-Wesley Publishing Company; 1982.

[5] Williams RL, Karacan I. Sleep disorders diagnosis and treatment. New York: John Wiley & Sons; 1978.

[6] Gould GA, Whyte KF, Rhind GB, et al. The sleep hypopnea syndrome. Am Rev Respir Dis 1998; 137:895–8.

[7] Moser NJ, Phillips BA, Berry DT, et al. What is hypopnea anyway? Chest 1994;105(2):426–8.

[8] Clinical Practice Review Committee. Position paper: hypopnea sleep disorders breathing in adults. Sleep 2001;24(4):469–70.

[9] A.A.S.M. Task Force. Sleep-related breathing disorders in adults. Recommendations for syndrome definition and measurement techniques in clinical research. Sleep 1999;22(5):667–89.

[10] Johnson PL, Edwards N, Burgess KR, et al. Detection of increased upper airway resistance during overnight polysomnography. Sleep 2005;28(1): 85–90.

[11] Ayappa I, Norman RG, Krieger AC, et al. Noninvasive detection of respiratory effort-related arousals (RERAs) by a nasal cannula/pressure transducer system. Sleep 2000;23(6):763–71.

[12] Bloom JW, Kaltenborn WT, Quan SF. Risk factors in a general population for snoring. Presented at Annual Meeting, American Thoracic Society. New Orleans, May 13, 1967.

S L E E P
M E D I C I N E
C L I N I C S

Sleep Med Clin 1 (2006) 461–463

Nonlaboratory Assessment of Sleep-Related Breathing Disorders

Michael Littner, MD[a],*, Max Hirshkowitz, PhD, D ABSM[b,c],
Amir Shararfkhaneh, MD, D ABSM[b,c], Sheila Goodnight-White, MD[b,c]

- Overview
- Pretest clinical assessment
- Cardiopulmonary recorder assessment
- Interpretation and disposition
- Summary
- References

At professional sleep society and pulmonary clinical meetings it has become fashionable to debate whether laboratory or nonlaboratory assessment should be used to diagnose sleep-related breathing disorders. The best approach involves integrating both approaches into a systematic evaluation program. Each technique has its own particular strengths and weakness, and, when combined in the proper manner, these work complementarily to the program's advantage.

In a previously published article on this topic the lead author reviewed evidence concerning standalone use of portable monitors in the patient's home [1]. Existing data were insufficient to support this approach, but it was concluded that with proper procedures and resources, portable cardiopulmonary sleep recording could provide a valuable addition to clinical sleep program (Fig. 1). These procedures and resources include

1. Proper patient selection
2. Use of an appropriate portable recorder

3. Interpretation of the portable recording by a qualified sleep specialist
4. Readily available access to laboratory polysomnography (when needed)
5. Systematic follow-up

Pretest clinical assessment

The first step in the process is to obtain from the patient the information needed to estimate the pretest probability for sleep-related breathing disorder. An assortment of questionnaires, symptom checklists, and calculations using anthropometric and self-reported data exist [2–5]. If clinical suspicion is high (or pretest probability exceeds 70%), the patient can be referred for portable study. If symptom presentation is mixed, the patient is not sleepy, or pretest probability is low, the patient should be referred for full laboratory assessment. Another reason to refer a patient for full laboratory assessment is the presence of signs or symptoms

a Veterans Administration Medical Center (111P), 16111 Plummer Street, Sepulveda, CA 91343, USA
b Baylor College of Medicine, 1 Baylor Plaza, Houston, TX 77030, USA
c Sleep Disorders & Research Center, Michael E. DeBakey Veterans Affairs Medical Center (111i), 2002 Holcombe Blvd., Houston, TX 77030, USA
* Corresponding author. Veterans Administration Medical Center (111P), Bldg. 200, Rm 3534, 16111 Plummer Street, Sepulveda, CA 91343.
E-mail address: mlittner@ucla.edu (M. Littner).

1556-407X/06/$ – see front matter © 2006 Elsevier Inc. All rights reserved.
sleep.theclinics.com

doi:10.1016/j.jsmc.2006.11.003

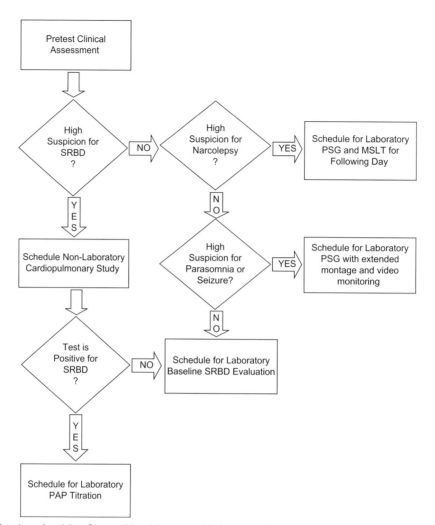

Fig. 1. Evaluation algorithm for combined home and laboratory sleep apnea program. Pretest probability for sleep apnea is determined, and if it is high, the patient is scheduled for nonlaboratory cardiopulmonary recorder sleep study. If the test is positive, patients are scheduled for positive airway pressure titration. If either the pretest probability for sleep apnea is low or a nonlaboratory study is negative, patients are schedule for attended laboratory overnight polysomnography as per current standards of practice.

suggesting additional, medically significant comorbid sleep disorders (eg, the patient bites his or her tongue at night and routinely sleepwalks). Nonetheless, in cases in which the sleep-related breathing disorder must be diagnosed and treated before the other conditions are addressed (eg, if there is a strong suspicion of sleep apnea but also some ancillary symptoms suggesting narcolepsy), one still might begin with a portable cardiopulmonary study.

Cardiopulmonary recorder assessment

The patient has a portable study; but the portable recorder must be competent. Portable monitors are classified as level II, III, and IV [6]. In this classification, as the level increases, the number of sleep and respiratory measures decreases. An unattended full polysomnographic recording with respiratory measurements and sleep staging constitutes a level II procedure. By contrast, level III involves three or more respiratory channels and heart rate (generally without sleep staging). These systems often are referred to as "cardiopulmonary recorders." When a system has only one or two channels (usually including oximetry), it falls into the level IV category. Currently, some level III cardiopulmonary recorders possess enough specificity to diagnose obstructive sleep apnea but lack adequate sensitivity to exclude obstructive sleep apnea when the overall study is negative.

Interpretation and disposition

An experienced sleep practitioner capable of evaluating both the clinical and the cardiopulmonary recorder information reviews the data. If the portable study is negative for sleep-disordered breathing, the patient is referred for an attended, in-laboratory, full polysomnographic diagnostic evaluation. A negative test does not rule out sleep-related breathing disorder. Cardiopulmonary recorders tend to underestimate severity, in part because central nervous system arousals typically are not scored because there is no electroencephalographic channel. Cardiopulmonary recorders readily detect gross pathophysiology in the form apnea episodes (complete or nearly complete cessations of breathing for 10 seconds or more). Competent recorders reliably distinguish hypopnea (shallow breathing) associated with oxyhemoglobin desaturation. However, more subtle respiratory events (eg, respiratory effort–related arousals) area not identified.

When the portable study is positive for obstructive sleep apnea, the patient is referred to the laboratory for titration using continuous positive airway pressure, bilevel positive airway pressure, or automatic self-adjusting positive airway pressure (if such a procedure is used in the sleep program). The use of automatic self-adjusting airway pressure for unattended titration is beyond the scope of this article; the reader is referred to the American Academy of Sleep Medicine evidence-based review and guidelines for further information [7,8].

Summary

Portable monitoring systems designed for nonlaboratory assessment of sleep-related breathing disorders are another tool available for practicing sleep medicine. Many of these level III devices are sleep cardiopulmonary recorders. These devices are not intended to replace polysomnography but rather to complement it when appropriate. When properly integrated into a sleep disorders program, nonlaboratory assessment can facilitate diagnosis of patients who have more severe sleep-disordered breathing. Thus, the next time you are asked to vote using your audience participation controller whether you think laboratory or nonlaboratory sleep recordings should be used to evaluate patients for sleep-disordered breathing, press both.

References

[1] Littner M. Portable monitoring in the diagnosis of the obstructive sleep apnea syndrome. Semin Respir Crit Care Med 2005;26:56–67.

[2] Netzer NC, Stoohs RA, Netzer CM, et al. Using the Berlin Questionnaire to identify patients at risk for the sleep apnea syndrome. Ann Intern Med 1999;131:485–536.

[3] Gurubhagavatula I, Maislin G, Pack AI. An algorithm to stratify sleep apnea risk in a sleep disorders clinic population. Am J Respir Crit Care Med 2001;164:1904–9.

[4] Flemons WW, Whitelaw WA, Brant R, et al. Likelihood ratios for a sleep apnea clinical prediction rule. Am J Respir Crit Care Med 1994;150:1279–85.

[5] Viner S, Szalai JP, Hoffstein V. Are history and physical examination a good screening test for sleep apnea? Ann Intern Med 1991;115:356–9.

[6] Chesson AL Jr, Berry RB, Pack A. Practice parameters for the use of portable monitoring devices in the investigation of suspected obstructive sleep apnea in adults. Sleep 2003;26:907–13.

[7] Berry RB, Parish JM, Hartse KM. The use of auto-titrating continuous positive airway pressure for treatment of adult obstructive sleep apnea. An American Academy of Sleep Medicine review. Sleep 2002;25:148–73.

[8] Littner M, Hirshkowitz M, Davila D, et al. Standards of Practice Committee of the American Academy of Sleep Medicine. Practice parameters for the use of auto-titrating continuous positive airway pressure devices for titrating pressures and treating adult patients with obstructive sleep apnea syndrome. An American Academy of Sleep Medicine report. Sleep 2002;25:143–7.

SLEEP
MEDICINE
CLINICS

Sleep Med Clin 1 (2006) 465–473

Economics of Home Monitoring

Nizar Suleman, MD[a], Max Hirshkowitz, PhD, D ABSM[a,b],*

- Overview
- Methods
  Construction of cost savings-excess model
  Validation of model (proof of concept)
- Results

- Discussion
- Summary
- Acknowledgments
- References

Obstructive sleep apnea (OSA) is characterized by cessation of breathing or airflow reduction during sleep. It affects approximately 4% of the middle-aged adult population [1]. Patients with undiagnosed OSA have considerably higher medical costs compared with those who do not have the condition, and it has been estimated that untreated sleep apnea may cause $3.4 billion in additional medical costs in the United States [2]. In the United States, the recommended method for diagnosing OSA is laboratory monitoring with attended polysomnography (PSG) [3]. Continuous positive airway pressure (CPAP) is currently a preferred treatment for OSA, but it requires titration while the patient sleeps in the laboratory. In patients with severe OSA, a split night protocol often is used. In a split night protocol, the first 2 to 3 hours are used for confirming the diagnosis, and the remainder of the night is used to titrate CPAP. In less severe cases, two laboratory studies are performed, the first for diagnosis, and the second for CPAP titration.

Portable sleep monitoring systems for diagnosing OSA are classified based on the complexity and number of parameters monitored [4]. Type two monitors record seven channels and are similar to devices used in attended PSG. Type three monitors typically record four channels, including airflow, oxygen saturation, heart rhythm, and respiratory effort but do not identify sleep stages.

The clinical demand for tests that diagnose possible sleep-disordered breathing is rising. This demand coupled with long waiting periods for sleep bed availability, especially in capitated health systems may lead to delays in diagnosing OSA. Portable, unattended cardiopulmonary recordings (CPRs) (type three monitors) are proposed as a lower cost alternative to laboratory PSG and as a means to improve timeliness of health care delivery for patients with OSA, especially in capitated health care systems that are oversubscribed and have limited resources. This claim, however, has neither been modeled nor empirically demonstrated. In contrast, it can be claimed that CPRs would lead to over testing and increased costs. Therefore, we undertook this study to determine the cost effectiveness of CPR based on data obtained from four different sleep centers. The four sources were a government hospital, a county hospital, a university-affiliated private hospital, and a free-standing private clinic. These settings differed markedly in population profiles and referral patterns.

[a] Baylor College of Medicine, 1 Baylor Plaza, Houston, TX 77030, USA
[b] Sleep Disorders & Research Center, Michael E. DeBakey Veterans Affairs Medical Center (111i), 2002 Holcombe Blvd., Houston, TX 77030, USA
* Corresponding author. Sleep Center (111i), 2002 Holcombe Blvd., Bldg. 100, Rm 6C344, Houston, Texas 77030.
E-mail address: maxh@bcm.tmc.edu (M. Hirshkowitz).

doi:10.1016/j.jsmc.2006.09.001

Methods

This study was performed in two phases.

1. Construction of model to estimate cost savings-excess of CPR to diagnose OSA in hypothetical populations with varying proportions of patients with an apnea plus hypopnea index (AHI) of 15 to 30, and using different cost ratios of CPR to PSG. AHI is the number of apnea and hypopnea episodes per hour of polysomnographically defined sleep.
2. Validation of model using data already collected from patients undergoing PSG for suspected OSA in four centers with different population profiles, severity patterns, and referral patterns.

Construction of cost savings-excess model

Depending on the severity of their AHI, patients with possible OSA undergoing PSG testing may (1) have a negative test result, (2) have a positive test result but not meet criteria early enough in the night to undergo CPAP titration and therefore have to return on another night, or (3) meet diagnostic criteria during the first 2 to 3 hours of the study and then have a CPAP titration during the remainder of the night (i.e., have a split-night study). Uncommonly, (4) a patient with suspected OSA will not sleep for an adequate amount of time in the laboratory during PSG monitoring, thereby resulting in an inconclusive study.

For purposes of this study, we stratified patients with suspected OSA into three categories based on the severity of their AHI: category A (AHI <15), category B (AHI 15 to 30), category C (AHI >30). Using this stratification and practice parameters for the indications for PSG in patients with suspected OSA [5], patients with suspected OSA who underwent PSG testing and followed standard-of-care practice would fall into the three categories as outlined in Table 1 (category A, negative PSG; category B, diagnostic PSG followed by a subsequent full-night titration; or category C, split night PSG). It is important to note that this classification is simplified and that overlap between the groups exists (eg, a patient with AHI 25 [category B by AHI number] during the first 2 hours of the PSG would meet criteria for split-night study but undergo a split-night study, whereas a patient with AHI 36 [category C by AHI number] who met diagnostic criteria late in the study and could not have a split-night study and would have to return to undergo CPAP titration).

In general, CPR devices are less sensitive than laboratory PSG for the diagnosis of OSA. One reason is electroencephalography is not usually measured; therefore, central nervous system arousals cannot be detected. Another reason is that AHI during CPR is calculated using the total time in bed as the denominator rather than total sleep time. Because time in bed must equal or exceed total sleep time, the larger denominator falsely lowers AHI and potentially can produce a false-negative test results. Therefore, a patient with suspected OSA who has a negative CPR study and a high pretest probability of OSA should have to undergo a laboratory PSG to rule out OSA. Table 1 also outlines testing that would be performed if CPRs were applied as a diagnostic tool in patients with suspected OSA. Again, patients are classified in categories, depending on AHI, and as in the standard-of-care pathway, significant overlap exists between the groups.

Thus, it can be seen that there is a potential for cost savings using CPR to diagnose OSA in patients with category B apnea, whereas there is a potential for cost excess arising from extra testing in patients with categories A and C. Using this model, and an equation for the net amount of cost savings-excess for each 100 patients with suspected OSA who have testing with standard of care or proposed CPR testing can be derived as follows:

$$NA = [y(C+2P)+z(C+P)+x(C+P)$$
$$+(1-x-y-z)(C+P)]$$
$$-[2yP+zP+2xP+P(1-x-y-z)]$$

$$= [yC+2yP+zC+zP+xC+xP+C-xC-yC$$
$$-zC+P-xP-yP-zP]-[2yP+zP+2xP+P$$
$$-xP-yP-zP]$$

$$= [yP+C+P]-[yP+xP+P]$$

$$= [c-xP]$$

NA can be multiplied for the number of patients that will be tested, to give a cost savings-excess for the population to be tested.

P = cost of PSG
C = cost of CPR
x = proportion of patients with category B OSA
y = proportion of patients with category A OSA and AHI 5 to 15, with symptoms
z = proportion of patients with category A OSA and AHI <15, without symptoms
NA = net amount of cost savings-excess for each patient with suspected OSA

A positive net amount represents excess cost of CPR; a negative net amount represents cost savings of CPR

Using varying cost ratios of CPR and PSG as well as different proportions of patients with Category B AHI in the population, a cost savings-excess model can be constructed (Fig. 1A). Using

Table 1:   **Proposed patient category and evaluation schedule**

Patient category	AHI/RDI	Standard of care	Proposed CPR pathway	Cost savings excess estimate for each group
C	AHI >30	P_{spl}	$C + P_{tit}$	C
B	RDI 15–30	$P_{bsl} + P_{tit}$	$C + P$	$P - C$
A	RDI <15 (no symptoms)	P	$C + P$	C
	RDI 5–15 (symptoms)	P + P	$C + P + P$	C

Abbreviations: P_{spl}, polysomnography (split night); P_{tit}, polysomnography (titration); P_{bsl}, polysomnography (baseline); C, cardiopulmnary recording study.

this model, a cost savings-excess per 100 patients with suspected OSA who are tested using either the standard-of-care pathway or the CPR pathway can be estimated. For example: using a CPR to PSG cost ratio of 1:2 (CPR is 50% the cost of PSG) and a cost of PSG as $1000, testing a patient population with 20% category B patients using the proposed CPR protocol would lead to a cost excess of $30,000 per 100 patients tested; a population with 50% class B patients would break even, and a population with 80% class B patients would save $30,000 per 100 patients tested with the CPR protocol. The break-even point and cost savings for various populations tested with CPR depends on the proportion of patients in a population with category B AHI as well as the cost ratio of CPR to PSG. As the cost of CPR decreases compared with PSG (i.e., the ratio of CPR to PSG decreases), the proportion of patients with category B AHI in a population needed for a cost break-even shifts toward zero. In general, as the proportion of patients in a population with category B AHI increases, there is a trend toward increasing cost savings when the CPR pathway is applied. However, break-even in cost of testing and cost savings using CPR pathway are achieved at higher proportions of category B patients and lower CPR to PSG ratios.

Similar models can be constructed using different costs of PSG. Another model using PSG cost of $650 is shown in Fig. 1B.

Thus, using a hypothetical population, known cost of PSG and CPR to PSG cost ratio, and assuming no overlap between the categories described above, it is possible to estimate a cost savings-excess amount if CPR is used to diagnose OSA in a specific population as well as theoretically identify which populations would incur a cost savings from using a CPR pathway for diagnosing OSA.

Validation of model (proof of concept)

We proceeded to validate the model, using laboratory PSG data already collected from four centers

with different population profiles and severity patterns.

Ideally, validation of this model would be done with a prospective randomized study, using CPR and PSG as diagnostic modalities for OSA. However, this study would be expensive and would use a diagnostic modality (CPR) for OSA, that has not been approved or recommended for routine use in nonattended settings. To overcome these barriers, we elected to validate the model using laboratory PSG data already collected as part of diagnostic workup for patients with suspected OSA.

Data collection for this study was performed using charts of patients who underwent laboratory PSG for suspected OSA. Consecutive patient charts were evaluated beginning on a set date and going backward until a total of 300 charts were included in each center.

Inclusion criteria

We reviewed charts of patients with suspected OSA who underwent attended laboratory PSG testing.

Exclusion criteria

Patients who were excluded from the review were those who (1) had a split night study but did not meet criteria for performing a split night study, (2) had incomplete data (answers to study-related questions, eg, Epworth Sleepiness Scale [ESS]), (3) had an inconclusive study (did not sleep in the laboratory for enough time), (4) had a titration PSG, but had no information on baseline study in the chart, and (5) had a titration study and had a baseline study that was done before the time frame in which data for 300 patient charts were collected for each center.

Data collected included type of test (split, baseline), date of test, date of birth, age, height, weight, body mass index (BMI), sex, ESS score (ESS), presence of self reported comorbid conditions, and other sleep-related non-OSA diagnoses.

Patients in each population were stratified according to the AHI measured during laboratory PSG. The AHI was based on frequency of overnight

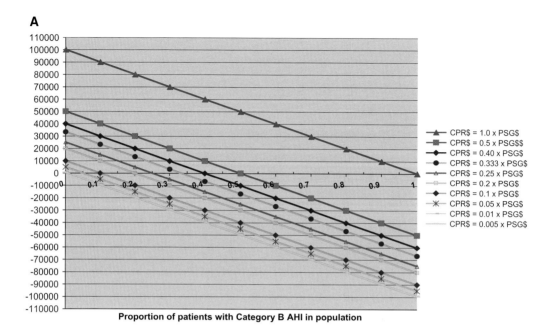

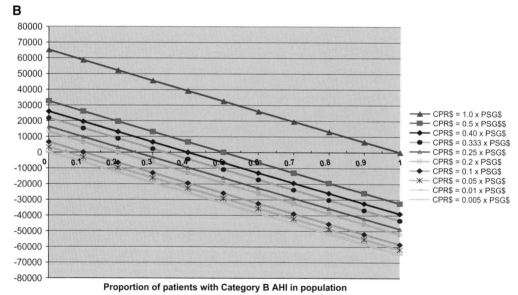

Fig. 1. (*A*) Cost savings-excess model based on varying proportions of patients with Class B AHI, using different cost ratios of CPR:PSG (assumes cost of PSG = $1000). (*B*) Cost savings-excess model based on varying proportions of patients with Class B AHI, using different cost ratios of CPR:PSG (assumes cost of PSG = $650).

events in those with baseline PSG and frequency of events in the first part of the study for those who had a split night study. The proportion of patients with category B AHI was determined from this stratification. Using this proportion, an "estimated" cost savings-excess figure was derived from the model (Fig. 2) based on a CPR to PSG cost ratio of 0.40 (from our market research).

Data from each patient (AHI and ESS) were reviewed and determination made as to where they

would fit regarding the diagnostic–treatment pathways described in Table 1. The purpose of reclassifying these patients into the three groups was to reduce the overlap between categories B and C as described above. Reclassifying these patients also simulated a "prospective" diagnostic trial. The proportion of patients who were now classified into category B AHI (patients in whom there would be a cost savings if CPR were to be used as a diagnostic tool, as from Table 1) was determined. This new proportion of

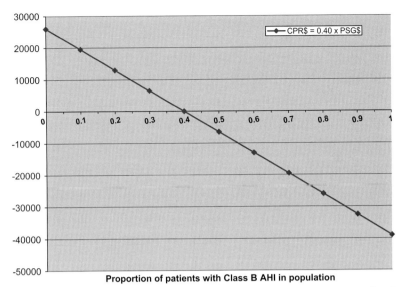

Fig. 2. Cost savings-excess model using cost of CPR as 40% of PSG (assumes cost of PSG = $650). Abbreviations: AHI, Apnea-hypopnea index; CPR$, cost of cardiopulmonary recording; PSG$, cost of attended laboratory polysomnography.

Category B AHI was used to determine an "expected" cost savings-excess from Fig. 2, thereby providing information to validate the model.

Results

A total of 1524 charts were reviewed for this study. A total of 1200 patient charts (300 in each center) were included for this study; 324 charts were excluded from the study based on exclusion criteria.

Table 2 summarizes the patient demographics, BMI, type of test, Apnea Index (AI) and AHI severity. Government (Veterans Affairs) patients were older and had a preponderance of male patients. County patients had a higher BMI and had a higher AHI severity of OSA. Private facilities tended to perform more baseline testing, probably because of the lower mean AHI in their populations. Table 3 summarizes the associated self-reported comorbidities, the percentage of patients with a diagnosis of OSA based on the report of PSG, and the percentages of non-OSA diagnoses. Hypertension was the most frequently associated comorbidity. In general, greater than 85% of patients having PSG for suspected OSA had the diagnosed confirmed, although in the Government population, this percentage was lower. However, there was a higher percentage of patients in the government population that had upper airway resistance syndrome.

Table 4A provides details on estimated and expected cost savings-excess for the different populations as well as the all populations as a group. For purposes of this study, we used a CPR to PSG

Table 2: **Demographic features of patient groups**

	GOV (n = 300)	COU (n = 300)	PUA (n = 300)	PFS (n = 300)	Total (n = 1200)
Study period	10/04-9/03	10/04-1/04	10/04-6/03	10/04-7/04	
Age	58.19 ± 11.44	49.48 ± 11.30	52.69 ± 13.16	49.20 ± 12.17	52.41 ± 12.56
Sex (M:F)	95:1	1:1.1	1.59:1	1.86:1	2.06:1
ESS	13.61 ± 5.75	13.71 ± 6.24	10.57 ± 5.72	11.29 ± 5.61	12.29 ± 6.01
BMI	33.47 ± 6.73	40.05 ± 10.50	32.76 ± 8.31	35.35 ± 22.94	35.40 ± 13.94
AI	23.7 ± 28.6	23.7 ± 48.9	8.72 ± 16.70	22.22 ± 32.03	19.55 ± 34.06
AHI	42.2 ± 34.8	61.8 ± 44.1	36.32 ± 33.20	36.40 ± 34.69	44.06 ± 38.39
Test type					
Baseline	128	104	169	197	598
Split	172	196	131	103	602

Abbreviations: COU, county; GOV, government; PUA, private university affiliated; PFS, private free standing; Total, all four groups.

Table 3: Associated comorbidities and diagnoses of patients undergoing PSG

	GOV (n = 300)	COU (n = 300)	PUA (n = 300)	PFS (n = 300)	TOTAL (n = 1200)
Associated comorbidity (%)					
DM	32.7	36.3	18.3	15.7	25.8
HTN	66.3	68.3	48.3	44.3	59.9
CVA	2.7	5.0	2.7	0.7	3.3
HT DX/CHF	28.0	27.3	17.0	7	19.8
COPD/LUNG DX	20	25.3	19.3	12.3	19.1
Depression	47.0	47.0	32.3	22.7	36.8
Diagnosis (%)					
OSA	80.0	90.3	87.0	92.0	87.4
PLMD (A)	25.0	11.7	19.0	6.7	15.7
PLMD (NA)	18.0	15.3	8.3	24.3	16.5
RLS	20.0	20.1	14.0	4.7	14.8
Sleep GERD	35.0	33.3	15.0	19.7	25.8
Dysom. Pain	10.7	4.7	9.0	0.7	6.3
Narcolepsy	1.3	0.3	0	0	0.4
Sleep bruxism	23.3	19.7	28.3	14.7	21.6
PPI	32.0	27.8	24.3	4.0	22.1
NLC	34.7	43.7	12.3	0.3	22.8
ISS	15.7	11.7	2.7	9.0	9.8
ISH	2.7	8.7	1.3	1.0	3.4
UARS	11.7	4	2.9	1.3	5
Primary snoring	3.0	2.7	4.3	4	3.5

Abbreviations: CHF, congestive heart failure; COPD, chronic obstructive pulmonary disease; COU, county; CVA, cerebro-vascular accident; DM, diabetes mellitus; GOV, government; HTN, hypertension; ISH, insufficient sleep hygiene; ISS, insufficient sleep syndrome; NLC, nocturnal leg cramps; PFS, private free standing; PLMD (A), periodic limb movement (arousing); PLMD (NA), periodic limb movement (nonarousing); PPI, psychophysiological insomnia; PUA, private university-affiliated; RLS, restless legs syndrome; Sleep GERD, sleep related gastroesophageal reflux disease; UARS, upper airway resistance syndrome.

ratio of 0.4, together with a PSG cost of $650. This was derived from an informal market survey. Application of CPR to diagnose OSA in all populations led to an increased cost of diagnosis when the populations were evaluated using their AHI profiles. However, when the same populations were re-evaluated after classifying patients according to their treatment status, all populations still showed cost excess of diagnosing OSA using CPR. The county patients even trended toward a higher cost excess. The private university-affiliated population showed a greater move toward break-even

Table 4A: Estimated and expected cost savings excess per 100 patients undergoing testing with CPR to evaluate suspected OSA

Population	Estimated cost-savings excess (%)		Expected cost savings excess (%)	
	B	$	B*	$**
GOV	17.3	$14755	25.3	$9100
COU	16.7	$15145	15.3	$16055
PUA	24.3	$10205	37.3	$1755
PFS	23.7	$10595	30.0	$6500
Overall	20.5	$12675	27.0	$8450

Given a CPR to PSG cost ratio of 0.40, and assuming PSG cost of $650. Positive value represents cost excess, negative value would represent cost savings; however, + values indicate additional costs.
Abbreviations: B, proportion of patients with category B AHI based on the AHI distribution; COU, county; GOV, government; PFS, private free standing; PUA, private university affiliated; $, estimated cost savings excess per 100 patients determined using B.
* Proportion of patients in category B after restratifying based on treatment diagnostic-treatment pathways.
** Expected cost savings excess per 100 patients determined using B*.

status probably based on a less severe AHI in that population.

Discussion

There is increasing awareness of OSA in the medical community as well as general population. Adequate access to facilities for the diagnosing OSA is still limited. Access remains a major barrier to providing care to these patients. It is estimated that OSA remains undiagnosed in at least 82% of men and 93% of women with the condition [6]. Several alternatives to overcome this barrier have been proposed, including use of portable home monitors/cardiopulmonary recording, empiric CPAP pressure prescription, as well as use of auto-titrating CPAP. However, all these modalities lack evidence from large, randomized, controlled trials and have been subject of major debate, especially on the use of portable home monitoring for diagnosing OSA. An argument for the use of CPR to diagnose OSA has been that it will provide an inexpensive means of diagnosing OSA; however, this claim has been neither modeled nor proven.

To our knowledge, this is the first study that has evaluated a cost savings-excess model that has incorporated split-night PSG as part of the diagnostic option in addition to using actual patient data to validate the model. This study shows that when using current costs of CPR and PSG as well as actual patient data, there is no significant cost benefit of applying CPR to diagnose OSA in patients with EDS. However, a break even can be realized if the cost ratio of CPR is dropped to 10% to 20% of the cost of PSG (using that cost ratio and the line plotted in Fig. 1, as well as the proportion of category B AHI patients in our study population in Table 4B). Fr there to be significant cost savings, the cost of CPR has to be lower than 5% to 10% of the current cost of PSG.

The lack of cost savings may be attributed to CPR, imposing an additional diagnostic step in patients with mild and severe OSA. Those with mild OSA will still need a laboratory PSG to rule out OSA. Patients with severe OSA would be diagnosed by home monitoring but then would require laboratory CPAP titration (both of which could be done in one night using a single split-night study).

The cost savings-excess model for this study was tested using data from a large population of patients who underwent PSG for suspected OSA and is representative of a broad spectrum of practice settings. This study was performed in one city, and results may not be generalized.

However, the large number of patients in each group as well as the patient diversity is a strong point for this study.

Although there is a trend toward cost savings in three of four population groups in this study, this trend does not lead to break-even or cost savings amounts. Even if a break-even point was to be realized using CPR, it would not justify replacing PSG with CPR because the two modalities are not equivalent. PSG has the further advantage of identifying non-OSA sleep-related disorders, especially limb movement disorders that often coexist with OSA. Failure to detect or treat these disorders when indicated would lead partial treatment of patients with EDS and necessitate further testing to elicit the cause of their symptoms.

In contrast, it has also been argued that PSG is not the "gold standard" for diagnosing OSA, partly because patients may not sleep as well in the sleep laboratory as they do at home and, in a minority of cases, not sleep at all. However, in most patients with suspected OSA, adequate recording times are achieved to make a diagnosis of OSA, and the patient then returns for another night of titration. A recent study found that the respiratory disturbance index (RDI) was similar in unattended home PSG and laboratory PSG, arguing against the fact that patients may not sleep as well in the sleep laboratory [7].

On the other hand, CPR tends to underestimate the RDI because the denominator for this index is based on time in bed, thus potentially leading to a negative test and need for laboratory PSG to definitively rule out OSA in a patient with EDS [11]. The diagnostic accuracy of CPR is also limited. Home unattended CPR may have a 22% to 37%

Table 4B: Estimated and expected cost savings excess of using to CPR to diagnose OSA, given a CPR: PSG cost ratio of 0.40

Class	GOV	COU	PUA	PFS	GLOBAL
AASM 10-30 Class, CPR$ = 20% PSG$					
Sample-based proportion of Class B	23.3%	20.3%	35.3%	33.0%	28.0%
Treatment-based proportion of Class B	24.7%	21.3%	25.0%	32.0%	25.8%
AASM 15-30 Class, CPR$ = 20% PSG$					
Sample based proportion of Class B	17.3%	16.7%	24.3%	23.7%	20.5%
Treatment based proportion of Class B	25.3%	15.3%	37.3%	30.0%	27.0%

indeterminate result rate as well as a misclassification rate of 5% to 16% [8]. These high rates have the potential to increase cost of testing (eg, PSG to definitively rule in or rule out OSA in indeterminate tests) and increase patient anxiety (unneeded treatment or no treatment for those misclassified). The model assumes an AHI threshold of 15 for a positive test for diagnosing CPR. An AHI threshold of 10 to 15 is common in studies evaluating CPR as a means to diagnose OSA. The mean AHI in most studies evaluating CPR was in the moderate-to-severe range (AHI >20); therefore, the results of these tests may not be generalizable to populations with lower severity of OSA [8]. Current data on CPR are also limited to studies performed in sleep centers that have a high pretest probability of OSA (ie, low false-negative rate) as well as inclusion of patients without significant comorbid illness such as lung disease, which can influence the performance of a monitor in which pulse oximetry plays a large role in event (apnea/hypopnea) definition [8].

An argument for the application of CPR for diagnosing OSA in patients with EDS can be made regarding overcoming the long waiting times for laboratory PSG bed space. However, once a patient has OSA diagnosed based on results of CPR, there is still considerable wait time to get CPAP titration. Auto-titrating CPAP has been proposed as an alternative to laboratory titration; however, data on this modality are limited.

This study has several limitations. First, it is not prospective. The model may be oversimplified by grouping together patients into classes based on the severity of their AHI. Another important assumption is the equivalence in cost between baseline and split-night studies in the model. This difference is minimal, and including it in the model makes it more complicated. The study also assumes that different CPR devices are similar in their sensitivities and costs. Validation studies of diagnostic methods for OSA have produced a broad spectrum of sensitivities and specificities using varying technologies and data handling approaches. Some investigators have used the term *diagnostic agreement* to determine the degree of diagnostic error between a CPR and PSG [9]. Diagnostic agreement is dependent on the level of AHI for a positive test, and values of 78.6% to 86.7% have been quoted.

The level of diagnostic agreement for CPR that was considered in this study is quite liberal. Selection of a higher AHI as a cutoff for positive test result in CPR would lead to an even higher number of false-negative results when patients have CPR testing, and therefore more frequent need for laboratory PSG to rule in or rule out OSA, and therefore extra testing. Less-expensive CPR devices can be used to achieve break-even status, but the diagnostic accuracy of these devices is even lower and the cost benefit not realizable.

This study does not take into consideration cost utility analysis or deal with quality-adjusted life-years as a result of earlier diagnosis and treatment of OSA. This analysis has been performed using a decision tree model that compares PSG, home testing, and empirical therapy [10]. Using a set of several variables including pretest probability of OSA, varying sensitivities and specificities of PSG and home testing, different costs of PSG and home testing, and the cost of office visits and health care costs of untreated OSA, the authors concluded that PSG provided improved quality-adjusted life 5 years after the initial evaluation over both home study and empiric therapy under most modeled conditions. The study did not take into consideration utility of split-night testing, which may be slightly more expensive than baseline testing but provides even more cost savings and may have provided greater cost savings. It is thought that performing a spit-night study compromises the usefulness of the study and may not achieve an adequate titration pressure because of time constraints [11]. But, when protocols for titration are used, most patients can be adequately titrated. In our study, a minority of patients who had a split-night study could not be titrated adequately.

Another consideration that was not directly addressed in this study is whether CPR used to diagnose OSA in the model was in the form of unattended or attended sleep monitoring. Reuveni and coworkers [12] developed and performed a cost effectiveness analysis comparing PSG, unattended home partial sleep monitoring (or CPR), and attended partial sleep monitoring. They concluded that unattended CPR was not cost effective when compared with PSG or attended CPR. The utility of split-night PSG was not considered in this analysis.

Data loss, as well as other sources of technical failure especially in unattended CPR studies, warrants repeat testing and increases cost of testing when CPR is used to diagnose OSA. A wide range of data loss as been reported [9,13–15].

The costs of PSG and CPR used in this study are based on estimated operational cost and informal market research. The overall diagnostic and operational costs in sleep laboratories are not well documented [10,16]. Knowledge of these costs, as well as consideration of regional difference, would increase the effectiveness of this model.

CPR does have the potential to reduce the costs of diagnosing OSA. This is dependent on the cost of CPR compared with PSG, a lower cost of PSG, and the proportion of patients with category B AHI (AHI 15-30) in the population (those in whom CPR would lead to a cost savings). A thorough evaluation of CPR with careful selection and standardization of specific device(s), as well as randomized controlled trials, need to be performed before incorporating it into routine clinical practice. When large randomized trials comparing different devices cannot be performed, development of models with greater complexity than the one we have described will provide more information to health care managers who might be tempted, on the basis of the high sensitivity and specificity of portable monitoring, to encourage use of this inexpensive method to diagnose OSA at a perceived lower cost. In the meantime, a more precise and more expensive test (PSG) not only provides better outcomes, but also represents a cost-effective option relative to portable home monitoring and empiric therapy.

Portable monitoring currently is recommended as an acceptable alternative in some clinical circumstances, including cases of severe clinical symptoms indicative of OSA in which PSG is not available; cases in which patients are unable to be studied in a sleep laboratory [4]; and follow-up studies for patients who have OSA diagnosed by PSG after therapy has been initiated. However, these circumstances are limited.

Summary

This study shows that the cost of studies to diagnose OSA can be modeled. When CPR is used as a tool to diagnose OSA in populations in different practice settings, a cost savings-excess amount can be projected based on the cost of PSG, CPR to PSG cost ratio, as well as the proportion of patients with an AHI 15 to 30 (category B) in the populations. CPR at its current cost does not provide a cost effective means to diagnose OSA; however, cost savings can be achieved if the cost of CPR is lower than 10–20% the cost of PSG.

Acknowledgments

The authors wish to thank Virginia Vasquez, Mischelle McFall, Brian Gaden, Cheryl May, and Ruth Lynn for their assistance with retrieving patient charts for this study. This paper is dedicated to my father.

References

[1] Pack A. An overview of obstructive sleep apnea: epidemiology, pathophysiology, clinical presentation, and treatment. Adv Intern Med 1994;39: 517–67.

[2] Kapur V, Blough DK, Sandblom RE, et al. The medical cost of undiagnosed sleep apnea. Sleep 1999;22:749–55.

[3] American Sleep Disorders Association. Practice parameters for the indications for polysomnography and related procedures: Polysomnography Task Force, American Sleep Disorders Association Standards of Practice committee. Sleep 1997;20: 406–22.

[4] Chesson AL, Berry RB, Pack A. Practice parameters for the use of portable monitoring devices in the investigation of suspected obstructive sleep apnea in adults. Sleep 2003;26:907–13.

[5] Kushida CA, Littner MR, Morgenthaler T, et al. Practice parameter for the indications for polysomnography and related procedures: an update for 2004. Sleep 2005; in press.

[6] Young T, Evans L, Finn L, et al. Estimation of the clinically diagnosed proportion of sleep apnea syndrome in middle-aged men and women. Sleep 1997;20:705–6.

[7] Iber C, Redline S, Gilpin AM, et al. Polysomnography performed in the unattended home versus that attended laboratory setting – Sleep Heart Health Study Methodology. Sleep 2004;27: 536–40.

[8] Flemons WW, Littner MR, Rowley JA, et al. Home diagnosis of sleep apnea: a systematic review of the literature. Chest 2003;124:1543–79.

[9] White DP, Gibb TJ, Wall JM, et al. Assessment of accuracy and analysis time of a novel device to monitor sleep and breathing in the home. Sleep 1995;18:115–26.

[10] Chervin RD, Murman MS, Malow BA, et al. Cost-utility of three approaches to the diagnosis of sleep apnea: polysomnography, home testing, and empirical therapy. Ann Intern Med 1999; 130:496–505.

[11] Chesson AL, Ferber RA, Fry JM, et al. The indications or polysomnography and related procedures. Sleep 1997;20:423–87.

[12] Reuveni H, Schweitzer E, Tarasiuk A. A cost-effectiveness analysis of alternative at-home or in-laboratory technologies for the diagnosis of obstructive sleep apnea syndrome. Med Decis Making 2001;21:451–8.

[13] Whittle AT, Finch SP, Mortimore IL, et al. Use of home sleep studies for diagnosis of sleep apnea/hypopnea syndrome. Thorax 1997;52: 1068–73.

[14] Zucconi M, Ferini-Strambi L, Castronov V, et al. An unattended device for sleep-related breathing disorders: validation study in suspected obstructive sleep apnea syndrome. Eur Resp J 1996;9: 1251–6.

[15] Ferber R, Milman R, Coppola M, et al. Portable recording in the assessment of obstructive sleep apnea: ASDA standards of practice. Sleep 1994; 17:378–92.

[16] Pack I, Gurubhagavatula I. Economic implications of the diagnosis of obstructive sleep apnea. Ann Intern Med 1999;130:533–4.

SLEEP
MEDICINE
CLINICS

Sleep Med Clin 1 (2006) 475–482

ELSEVIER
SAUNDERS

Upper Airway Resistance Syndrome

Kanta Velamuri, MD[a,b],*

- Definition
- Clinical features
  Epidemiology
  Symptoms
  Signs
  Sleep architecture
- Pathophysiology
- Diagnosis
  Polysomnographic findings
  Increased respiratory effort

- Differential diagnosis
- Treatment
  Weight loss
  Positive airway pressure
  Oral appliances
  Surgery
  Other approaches
- Consequences and prognosis
- Summary
- References

Obstructive sleep apnea syndrome (OSAS), obstructive sleep hypopnea syndrome (OSHS), and idiopathic hypersomnia are well-known sleep disorders associated with excessive daytime sleepiness. Upper airway resistance syndrome (UARS) is a lesser-known sleep disorder. First described in 1993 by Guilleminault and colleagues [1], UARS is a diagnosis considered in patients who have excessive daytime sleepiness but lack the typical findings of apnea and hypopnea on polysomnographic evaluation. Although some experts doubt whether UARS is a distinct disorder, more and more evidence points to its being a separate entity with features distinct from OSAS and OSHS. Knowledge and awareness of UARS have increased in the past decade, but there is much to be learned about the syndrome.

Definition

Essential features in the diagnosis of UARS include

1. Excessive daytime sleepiness/daytime fatigue
2. Polysomnographic findings of an apnea/hypopnea index of less than 5 per hour of sleep

3. Elevated electroencephalographic (EEG) arousal index (>10 EEG arousals/hour) associated with increased respiratory efforts

Supportive features to the diagnosis include a history of snoring, a pattern of increasing snoring (crescendo snoring) before EEG arousal, and clinical improvement with nasal continuous positive airway pressure (CPAP) therapy [2].

Clinical features

Epidemiology

The prevalence of UARS is estimated at 8.4% of all patients referred for sleep-disordered breathing. UARS, however, is an underrecognized syndrome with atypical features. Therefore, it is possible that a majority of patients are never even referred to a clinical sleep laboratory for evaluation.

UARS is seen in younger age groups than is obstructive sleep apnea (OSA). In fact, in children UARS is more common than OSA among patients referred for evaluation of sleep-disordered

[a] Pulmonary Medicine, Sleep Disorders and Research Center, Michael E. DeBakey Veterans Affairs Medical Center (111i), 2002 Holcombe Blvd., Houston, TX 77030, USA
[b] Section of Pulmonary and Critical Care Medicine, Baylor College of Medicine, 1 Baylor Plaza BCM 620, Houston, TX 77030, USA
* Correspondence. MED VAMC Pulmonary Medicine (111i), 2002 Holcombe Blvd., Houston, TX 77030.

doi:10.1016/j.jsmc.2006.10.004

breathing [3]. The male predominance noted in OSA is not seen in UARS: a more equal distribution between sexes is seen. UARS also is seen in patients who have a lower body mass index (BMI).

Symptoms

Daytime fatigue and excessive daytime sleepiness

Patients who have OSA and UARS have similar symptoms of excessive daytime fatigue and sleepiness. In a study comparing 12 patients with UARS to 12 patients each with OSA and OSHS and 12 matched normal controls, patients with UARS were as sleepy as patients with OSA and OSHS compared to the normal subjects (Epworth Sleepiness Scale score mean, 11.9 in UARS group and 12.4 and 12.6 in the OSA group and OSHS group, respectively, compared to 3.8 in normal controls). Mean sleep latency on the Multiple Sleep Latency Test (MLST), an objective measure of sleepiness, also showed similar results in the groups of patients who had sleep-related breathing disorders: 8 minutes in UARS and 7.9 minutes in OSA, compared with 16.8 minutes in controls [4].

Snoring

Snoring was thought to be an essential feature of UARS. In the original report by Guilleminault, snoring was present in 100% of the men and 75% of the women studied [1]. Subsequent studies found that patients who have UARS may present without snoring. About 9% of patients who have UARS have silent UARS [5].

Insomnia

Patients who have UARS also may present with insomnia or poor-quality nighttime sleep. Guilleminault and colleagues [6] studied a cohort of 394 postmenopausal women who had a complaint of insomnia. Seventy percent of these women had sleep-disordered breathing; 15.7% had UARS. Among these patients, those treated for sleep-disordered breathing had better improvement of symptoms than those treated for insomnia [7].

Functional and somatic symptoms

Patients who have UARS frequently present with symptoms similar to functional somatic syndromes (eg, chronic fatigue syndrome, fibromyalgia, irritable bowel syndrome, and migraine/tension headaches). Other symptoms include insomnia, nonrefreshing sleep, heartburn, headaches, depression, and orthostatic syncope [8].

Pediatric symptoms

The pediatric population with UARS differs from adults with UARS in their presenting clinical symptoms. Sleepwalking, night terrors, disturbed nocturnal sleep, abnormal shyness, and rebellious and aggressive behavior are common symptoms in children who have UARS [3].

Signs

Certain orocraniofacial features are closely associated with UARS, especially in children. These features include a small triangular chin, a steep mandibular plane, retroposition of the mandible, a long face, a high hard palate, and an elongated soft palate. Cephalometrics may reveal small posterior airway space.

Sleep architecture

The total sleep time (TST) of patients with UARS is significantly less than normal but more than that of patients with OSA. Patients with OSA have more episodes of waking after sleep onset than do patients with UARS resulting in a lower TST. There is no significant difference in stage 1 and 2 non–rapid eye movement (NREM) sleep in patients who have UARS, but the total percentage of time in slow-wave sleep (SWS) and rapid eye movement (REM) sleep is lower than normative values. When compared to patients with OSA, patients with UARS spend more time in SWS.

Polysomnograms of some patients who have UARS show a pattern of alpha-delta sleep. This pattern is marked by an intrusion of alpha waves into an overall SWS pattern. Alpha-delta sleep also is seen in functional somatic syndromes. Spectral power analysis shows that patients who have UARS have normal-appearing SWS but less total SWS, a higher absolute delta power in NREM sleep with loss of normal decrement, and a significantly higher power density in the alpha and beta bandwidths than do controls [4]. It has been postulated that abnormal inspiratory efforts lead to a higher amount of alpha frequency in patients who have UARS; the increased amount of alpha frequency signifies a heightened vigilance, which may explain why patients with UARS do not have complete airway closure and desaturations like patients with OSA do. The increased alpha and delta power also may explain the symptoms of daytime sleepiness and tiredness in patients who have UARS.

Pathophysiology

Much of the knowledge of the pathophysiology of UARS is based on studies on normal subjects and subjects who have OSA.

In normal subjects, there is a decrease in genioglossus activity as well as the activity of the tensor palatini muscle during sleep. This decreased activity makes the tongue and soft palate relax and tend to fall backward, narrowing the pharyngeal airway and increasing the supraglottic resistance. In normal subjects, however, airway occlusion does not occur because the neuromuscular force of the pharyngeal dilating muscles prevents the airway from collapsing [9].

In patients who have sleep-disordered breathing, however, this normal balance is disrupted by two main factors: abnormal airway anatomy and abnormal airway function.

Patients who have OSAS have been shown to have a lower total pharyngeal area resulting from subtle anatomic changes or from obvious anatomic features such as micrognathia, macroglossia, or tonsillar/adenoidal hypertrophy [10]. In UARS, as well, certain orofacial features are more common, including a small triangular chin, a steep mandibular plane, retroposition of the mandible, a long face, a high hard palate, and an elongated soft palate. This abnormal airway anatomy in patients who have UARS and OSAS/OSHS predisposes toward airway collapse [11].

In addition to abnormal anatomy, patients who have UARS and OSAS/OSHS have been found to have abnormal airway function. One important abnormality is an increase in the collapsibility of pharyngeal wall. This collapsibility has been defined as the critical pressure (Pcrit) surrounding the collapsible part of the pharyngeal airway. In normal subjects, the Pcrit is always negative, thus preventing airway collapse. In patients who have OSAS/OSHS, the critical pressure is less negative and is often positive, predisposing to airway collapse. Gold and colleagues [12] measured the Pcrit in normal subjects, in patients who had UARS, and in patients who had OSA/OSHS. They found a mean Pcrit $\pm$ SD of -15.4 ± 6.1 cm H_2O in normal patients, -4 ± 2.1 cm H_2O in patients who had UARS, -1.6 ± 2.6 cm H_2O in patients who had mild OSAS/OSHS, and 2.4 ± 2.8 cm H_2O in patients who had severe OSAS/OSHS.

Another abnormal function seen in OSA is a failure of reflex activation of the pharyngeal dilator muscles in response to airway occlusion. Patients who have OSAS have evidence of neurogenic lesions in the palatopharyngeal muscles on biopsy and abnormal sensory input because of these lesions. In a study with two-point palatal discrimination, patients who had OSAS had a clear impairment of their palatal sensory input [13]. This disruption of sensory input results in the forces of abnormal anatomy and increased collapsibility leading to airway occlusion. This airway occlusion leads to airflow limitation and desaturations and eventually arousal.

Patients who have UARS differ from patients who have OSAS/OSHS in this regard. Patients who have UARS have an intact and heightened response to airway occlusion. Two-point palatal discrimination in patients who have UARS is similar to that of normal subjects [13]. This response leads to increased respiratory effort and arousals. The higher alpha frequency seen in patients who have UARS may result from this heightened vigilance of the brain to the occlusive events and a constant effort to keep the airways patent. Therefore in patients who have UARS, no apneic or hypopneic episodes or desaturations are seen.

Patients who have UARS have an increase in arousals. Repetitive short arousals from any cause have been shown to cause increased daytime sleepiness and increased arousal threshold (an important defense mechanism) toward the latter third of the night [14]. Respiratory-associated arousals may have different physiologic effects than non-respiratory arousals (eg, auditory-induced arousals) [15]. The arousals in UARS lead to significant sleep fragmentation and symptoms of daytime sleepiness.

Diagnosis

The diagnosis of UARS requires exclusion of OSAS/OSHS, demonstration of excessive daytime sleepiness, and evidence of sleep disruption due to flow limitation and increased respiratory effort.

Polysomnographic findings

Standard polysomnography is used to demonstrate sleep disruption. In patients who have UARS, polysomnography shows repetitive alpha arousal lasting longer than 10 seconds. These arousals are called respiratory effort-related arousals (RERAs). A RERA is an abnormal breathing event characterized by increased respiratory effort that leads to an arousal from sleep but does not meet the criteria for hypopnea or apnea. Diagnosis of UARS requires more than five RERAs per hour of sleep. Also seen are repetitive microarousals lasting 3 to 10 seconds, increases in snoring just before the arousal, increases in inspiratory time and decrease in expiratory time. No apneas, hypopneas, or changes in arterial oxygen saturation are seen.

Limitation in airflow and increased upper airway resistance are also seen on the polysomnograms of patients with UARS. Upper airway resistance can be measured using direct pressure feedback from patients wearing tightfitting full-face masks to measure tidal volume. These masks, however, tend to disturb sleep quality. An alternative method for measuring airflow uses a nasal cannula attached to a sensitive pressure transducer. The transducer detects the pressure fluctuations caused by inspiration and expiration that are proportional to flow. This method gives measurements in airflow comparable to a pneumotachograph without the intrusive tight facemask. A flattened flow/time contour or a plateau on the inspiratory waveform corresponds to increased airway resistance and esophageal pressure swings [16].

Increased respiratory effort

Currently, the standard for the measurement of respiratory effort is esophageal pressure (Pes) monitoring [17]. Pes monitoring can be done by many different techniques. One method for esophageal manometry uses an esophageal balloon, about 3.2 cm in circumference, attached to a long polyethylene catheter that is connected to a pressure transducer. The balloon is positioned in the mid-esophagus. Advantages of this technique are reduced cardiographic artifact; disadvantages include the potential for holes, improper placement, incorrect volume of air in the balloon, and dislodgment. Another technique for monitoring Pes is by using a fluid-filled catheter system similar to the system used to monitor arterial pressure in ICUs. This system uses a high-pressure, low-flow valve that is connected to the pressure transducer and catheter (pediatric, 6-F nasogastric tube). A pressure infuser keeps a pressure of 300 mm Hg on a saline bag. The fluid in the catheter transmits pressure to the transducer and measures relative changes in Pes during sleep [18]. Advantages of this technique include tolerability, the small amount of fluid administered to patient, and simplicity of use. Chervin and Aldrich [19] evaluated the effect of this technique of esophageal manometry on sleep architecture. One hundred fifty-five patients who had Pes monitoring along with polysomnography were matched with comparison subjects who had similar apnea-hypopnea indices (AHI), minimum oxygen saturation, age, and sex who had undergone only polysomnography. Sleep architecture in the two groups was similar, with only small differences in total sleep time, latency to REM sleep, and other factors. MLSTs done the next day showed no differences between the groups, indicating that any disruption of sleep was not clinically significant. A third technique for measuring esophageal pressure changes is through a miniature pressure transducer at the end of a flexible polyurethane tube inserted in mid-esophagus. This technique is extremely precise but expensive.

Esophageal tracing patterns in upper airway resistance syndrome

Change in esophageal pressure (ΔPes) is measured by the peak–trough difference in the waveform on a breath–breath basis. A ΔPes less than 10 is within normal limits. The absolute negative nadir is also measured. A value of less than -10 cm H_2O is considered normal, although this parameter has not been well validated.

In UARS, the Pes tracing shows different patterns. One pattern is successively decreasing Pes with each breath, with the most negative nadir occurring one to two breaths before the arousal. This crescendo pattern occurs mainly in stage 1 and 2 NREM sleep. Another pattern shows regular decreased Pes (as compared with resting baseline), indicating a high respiratory effort. This pattern is seen mainly in SWS [20]. Both patterns show a reversal of the Pes nadir during and after the arousal. The Pes nadir becomes less negative than the breaths before the arousal. This reversal is important for distinguishing the increase in effort from tonic increases that can occur in stage 3 and 4 NREM. Although the values of the Pes nadir have been found to range between -17 and -68 cm H_2O, there is no absolute value of Pes nadir known to be abnormal.

Concerns regarding the validity of measurement (eg, possibility of stenting the airway open by the catheter, impairment of arousal responses by the local anesthesia used), patient refusal, and cost of monitoring have resulted in direct measurement of esophageal pressure being used in very few specialized centers. Many centers have tried to identify less invasive methods to measure respiratory effort.

Alternative methods to measure respiratory effort

Quantitative respiratory inductive plethysmography measurement detects changes in the volume of chest and abdomen over a breathing cycle. Asynchrony between chest and abdominal measurements has been shown to correspond to detection of hypopneas [21]. In a study evaluating this method in detecting UARS, a sensitivity of 67% and a specificity of 80% was obtained in overall stage 2 sleep [22]. For breaths immediately before arousals, however, respiratory inductance plethysmography had a better diagnostic accuracy, with 100% sensitivity and specificity. Therefore, the use of respiratory inductance plethysmography with a technique of analyzing the breaths before arousals is useful for noninvasively distinguishing patients who have UARS from those who do not.

Diaphragmatic electromyography indirectly measures respiratory effort based on surface electromyographic measurement of diaphragmatic movement.

Disadvantages of these two methods include changes in signal with change in body position and variation in signal caused by obesity.

Measurement of snoring amplitude and pattern of snoring was evaluated as an alternate measure of respiratory effort. A small study, however, showed no correlation with esophageal pressure [23].

Decreases in blood pressure measured by noninvasive beat-to-beat blood pressure monitors have been shown to correlate well with the degree of respiratory effort and increases in blood pressure with arousals.

Pulse transit time is the time required for the arterial pulse pressure wave to travel to the periphery from the aortic valve. Because the major determinant of pulse transit time is the blood pressure, it is a simpler method of detecting respiratory effort in sleep-related breathing disorders [24]. It is measured as the time between the R-wave on the ECG and the arrival of pulse wave at the finger. Pulse transit time is inversely proportional to blood pressure. A decrease in the pulse transit time measures arousals, and increases in PTT measure increased effort. A PTT tracing showing progressively increasing PTT ending in a decreased PTT (arousal) is seen in OSA. A study evaluating the value of pulse transit time in nonapneic respiratory events in nine patients who had mild-to-moderate sleep apnea showed a sensitivity of 79.9% and a positive predictive value of 91% using Pes as the gold standard [25]. This method, however, is fraught with problems of interobserver variability and undersampling errors.

Differential diagnosis

Obstructive sleep apnea

The main feature distinguishing UARS from OSA is included in its definition, namely, an AHI of less than 5. In BMI-matched patients who had OSA and UARS, the mean AHI was 33 in the OSA group and 2.8 in the UARS group. There are other differences between the two disorders, including the gender and age distribution, presenting symptoms, and other polysomnographic findings. Although OSA syndromes and UARS have many different clinical features, there are many similarities as well. Loube and Andrada [26] compared the respiratory polysomnographic parameters of 15 patients diagnosed as having UARS with a gender- and BMI-matched cohort of patients who had OSA. They found similar respiratory disturbance indices (when RERAs were included in the respiratory distress index), similar Pes nadir values, and the same degree of oxygen desaturations as measured by pulse oximetry.

Idiopathic hypersomnia

Idiopathic hypersomnia is a disorder characterized by chronic sleepiness without cataplexy that significantly impairs daytime performance. Clinically, patients who have idiopathic hypersomnia and patients who have UARS may describe symptoms of isolated excessive day sleepiness. Before a patient can be diagnosed as having idiopathic hypersomnia, a polysomnogram with Pes monitoring is essential to exclude patients who have UARS.

Periodic limb movements

Periodic limb movements in sleep (PLMS) is a syndrome in which repetitive stereotyped movements of one or both lower extremities occur during sleep. A study of 20 patients diagnosed as having PLMS showed the presence of RERAs in addition to the PLMs in 70% of patients. Sixty-three percent of all RERAs were associated with a limb movement. This association may explain why some patients who have PLMS have daytime sleepiness and do not improve with treatment with dopaminergic agents alone [27]

Nocturnal asthma

Patients who have UARS and those who have OSA describe symptoms of frequent nocturnal awakenings, poor sleep, and daytime sleepiness. A case report describes a 33-year-old woman with severe persistent asthma whose poorly controlled symptoms persisted despite an intensive regimen of oral steroids, inhaled bronchodilators, and steroids and methotrexate [28]. During a laryngoscopy done to assess for vocal cord dysfunction, retrolingual enlargement was seen. Polysomnography revealed no OSA. Because the patient did describe symptoms of excessive daytime sleepiness, frequent nocturnal awakenings, and snoring, a repeat polysomnography was done with an esophageal manometer. The patient was diagnosed as having UARS, and symptoms improved with treatment.

Treatment

The overall goal of treatment of sleep-related breathing disorders is to relieve symptoms, reduce morbidity and mortality, and, equally importantly, to improve the quality of life.

Weight loss

Although weight loss has been well studied in the treatment of OSA, there are no data regarding the benefit of weight loss in the treatment of UARS.

Positive airway pressure

In their initial report of UARS, Guilleminault and coworkers showed that CPAP treatment improved the symptoms and sleep of patients who had UARS [1]. After the initial report, CPAP was the only modality used in the treatment of UARS until around 1995. After 1995, CPAP is still the most frequently recommended treatment option, although other options such as dental devices, surgery, and radiofrequency treatment are recommended to some patients. There is an overall 19% noncompliance rate among CPAP users. Among compliant patients, CPAP treatment improves clinical symptoms and sleep macrostructure. Studies have shown improvement in the microstructure of sleep as well. Watanabe and colleagues [29] reported a small case series of patients who had UARS. Half of the patients agreed to try CPAP, and 57% continued with treatment. Those retreated with CPAP showed improvement in the Pes nadir and EEG arousal index. The main difficulties with the use of CPAP in the treatment on UARS is patient non-compliance and insurance refusal to cover treatment.

Oral appliances

Oral appliances are devices inserted into the mouth and used to modify the position of the mandible, the tongue, and or other structures in the upper airway. There are two types of oral appliances: mandibular-advancing devices and tongue-retaining devices. There are no randomized studies on the use of oral appliances in UARS. Yoshida [30] reported the use of oral appliances in 32 patients diagnosed as having UARS. All patients showed improvement in Epworth Sleepiness Scale scores, MSLT scores, arousal index, and minimal oxygen saturation values. No side effects were reported.

Surgery

The role of surgery in the management of UARS is not yet supported by good, randomized, controlled trials. Most of the studies done so far are either non-randomized or have other problems in methodology [31]. The first report of surgery in the treatment of UARS was in 1994. Forty-four patients who had UARS were treated with laser-assisted uvulopalatoplasty. Improvement in symptoms was reported in all these patients [32]. Another study described nine patients diagnosed as having UARS who were treated with upper airway surgery (septoplasty with turbinate reduction, laser-assisted uvulopalatoplasty, uvulopalatopharyngoplasty, mandibular osteotomy with tongue advancement, and hyoid myotomy with suspension). Three to 5 months after surgery, all patients had improved snoring and a significant decrease in their Epworth Sleepiness Scale scores. Two patients who underwent postoperative polysomnography with Pes monitoring showed a decrease in Pes nadir and respiratory distress index and improvement in lowest oxygen saturation [33].

Other approaches

Lofaso and colleagues [34] evaluated the effect of 7 days of zopiclone, a cyclopyrrolone hypnotic drug, on ventilation, sleep parameters, and daytime alertness in eight patients who had UARS. There was an improvement of sleep efficiency and average score on the MSLT in patients treated with zopiclone as opposed to those receiving placebo. The medication had no effect on sleep architecture, arousal index, or respiratory parameters.

Radiofrequency thermal ablation involves passing an electrical current through an electrode to induce a thermal lesion. This technique has been applied to the upper airway in patients who have sleep-disordered breathing. More work is needed to determine the ideal patients and the optimal methods for this procedure [35].

Consequences and prognosis

OSA is well known to cause serious cardiovascular complications. Not much is known, however, about the long-term consequences of UARS. Given the many similarities between the two conditions, it is reasonable to assume that the consequences are similar.

Sleep fragmentation, sleep restriction, and sleep deprivation generally lead to arterial hypertension. Recurrent hypoxemia and hypercarbia increase chemoreceptor firing, leading to increased sympathetic nerve activity and increases in arterial blood pressure. Arousals during sleep also directly activate the sympathetic nervous system and lead to a pressor response. A study of seven patients who had UARS and normal blood pressure showed progressive changes in ventricular size and a leftward shift of the interventricular septum related to the degree of respiratory efforts. These shifts were intermittent and occurred at Pes nadirs of more than -35 cm H_2O. Also seen were effort-related changes in blood pressure and spikes in blood pressure with each alpha arousal. This observation showed that, in patients who have UARS, stimulation of the sympathetic tone occurs similar to that seen in OSA, despite the absence of significant desaturations. In the same study, ambulatory blood pressure monitoring was done on a group of seven patients who had UARS and borderline hypertension. The blood pressure monitoring was done before treatment and then was repeated after 1 month of home CPAP therapy. The average daytime diastolic and systolic blood pressure recordings decreased significantly with therapy. The change in nighttime systolic blood pressure was not significant, but the nighttime diastolic blood pressure showed a significant decrease [36].

More recently, Guilleminault and colleagues [37] reported the natural evolution of UARS. In a prospective study, they attempted to contact all patients who had been diagnosed as having UARS in their sleep center between 1995 and 1998. Of the 138 patients identified, they contacted 105, and 94 agreed to participate. They underwent a follow-up visit and polysomnography. The study showed that none of the patients who came for follow-up were treated with nasal CPAP, mainly because their insurance companies refused to supply the machine. In fact, of the overall cohort of 138 patients, only 3 patients reported on the telephone that they were using nasal CPAP and had seen a clear improvement in their symptoms.

In follow-up all 94 patients described persistence of sleep-related symptoms, and the frequency of complaints had increased significantly over time. The highest increases were in symptoms of fatigue, insomnia, and depression. These patients also had increased use of hypnotic and antidepressant medications to treat their sleep symptoms (87.2% as opposed to 16% during the initial evaluation). Clinical interviews showed no significant changes in blood pressure or in cardiovascular or neurologic status. Repeat polysomnography showed findings similar to the initial polysomnogram. Only four patients had progressed to frank OSA, but these patients also had had a significant increase in BMI [37].

Summary

UARS is an important variant in the spectrum of sleep-related breathing disorders. Although not as obvious as sleep apnea in terms of symptoms, pathophysiology, and diagnosis, it frequently is the cause of excessive daytime sleepiness and fatigue and other long-term sequelae. Further research is required to improve understanding all aspects of this disorder.

References

[1] Guilleminault C, Stoohs R, Clerk A, et al. A cause of excessive daytime sleepiness: the upper airway resistance syndrome. Chest 1993;104:781–7.

[2] Wheatley JR. Definition and diagnosis of upper airway resistance syndrome. Sleep 2000;(Suppl 4): S193–6.

[3] Guilleminault C, Pelayo R, Leger D, et al. Recognition of sleep-disordered breathing in children. Pediatrics 1996;98:871–82.

[4] Guilleminault C, Do Kim Y, Chowdhuri S, et al. Sleep and daytime sleepiness in upper airway resistance syndrome compared to obstructive sleep apnoea syndrome. Eur Respir J 2001;17:838–47.

[5] Kristo DA, Lettieri CJ, Andrada T, et al. Silent upper airway resistance syndrome. Prevalence in a mixed military population. Chest 2005;127(5):1654–7.

[6] Guilleminault C, Palombini L, Poyares D, et al. Chronic insomnia, postmenopausal women, and sleep disordered breathing. Part 1. J Psychosom Res 2002;53:611–5.

[7] Guilleminault C, Palombini L, Poyares D, et al. Chronic insomnia, postmenopausal women, and sleep disordered breathing. Part 2. J Psychosom Res 2002;53:617–23.

[8] Gold AR, Dipalo F, Gold MS, et al. The symptoms and signs of upper airway resistance syndrome— a link to functional somatic syndromes. Chest 2003;123:87–95.

[9] Hoffstein V. How and why should we stabilize the upper airway? Sleep 1996;(9):S57–60.

[10] Kushida CA, Efron B, Guilleminault C. A predictive morphometric model for the obstructive sleep apnea syndrome. Ann Intern Med 1997; 127:581–7.

[11] Jamieson A, Guilleminault C, Partinen M, et al. Obstructive sleep apneic patients have craniomandibular abnormalities. Sleep 1986;9:469–77.

[12] Gold AR, Marcus CL, Dipalo F, et al. Upper airway collapsibility during sleep in upper airway resistance syndrome. Chest 2002;121(5):1531–40.

[13] Guilleminault C, Li K, Chen NH, et al. Two point palatal discrimination in patients with upper airway resistance syndrome, obstructive sleep apnea syndrome and normal controls. Chest 2002;122:866–70.

[14] Philip P, Stoohs R, Guilleminault C. Sleep fragmentation in normals: a model for sleepiness associated with upper airway resistance syndrome. Sleep 1994;17(3):242–7.

[15] Brooks D, Horner RL, Kozar LF, et al. Obstructive sleep apnea as a cause of systemic hypertension: evidence from a canine model. J Clin Invest 1997;99:106–9.

[16] Hosselet JJ, Norman RG, Ayappa I, et al. Detection of flow limitation with a nasal cannula/ pressure transducer system. Am J Respir Crit Care Med 1998;157:1461–7.

[17] American Academy of Sleep Medicine Task Force. Sleep-related breathing disorders in adults: recommendations for syndrome definition and measurement techniques in clinical research. Sleep 1999;22(5):667–89.

[18] Kushida CA, Giacomini A, Lee MK, et al. Technical protocol for the use of esophageal manometry in the diagnosis of sleep-related breathing disorders. Sleep Med 2002;3:163–73.

[19] Chervin RD, Aldrich MS. Effects of esophageal pressure monitoring on sleep architecture. Am J Respir Crit Care Med 1997;156:881–5.

[20] Guilleminault C, Poyares D, Palombini L, et al. Variability of respiratory effort in relation to sleep stages in normal controls and upper airway resistance syndrome patients. Sleep Med 2001; 2(5):397–405.

[21] Cantineau JP, Escourrou P, Sartene R, et al. Accuracy of respiratory inductive plethysmography during wakefulness and sleep in patients with obstructive sleep apnea. Chest 1992;102: 1145–51.

[22] Loube DI, Andrada T, Howard RS. Accuracy of respiratory inductive plethysmography for the diagnosis of upper airway resistance syndrome. Chest 1999;115:1333–7.

[23] Loewy D, Guilleminault C, Kushida CA. Prediction of esophageal pressure elevations by crescendo snoring patterns. Sleep 2000;23(Supp2):A7.

[24] Pitson DJ, Sandel A, Van den Hout R, et al. Use of pulse transit time as a measure of inspiratory effort in patients with obstructive sleep apnoea. Eur Respir J 1995;8:1669–74.

[25] Argod J, Pepin JL, Smith RP, et al. Comparison of esophageal pressure with pulse transit time as a measure of respiratory effort for scoring obstructive non-apneic respiratory events. Am J Respir Crit Care Med 2000;162:87–93.

[26] Loube DI, Andrada TF. Comparison of respiratory polysomnographic parameters in matched cohorts of upper airway resistance and obstructive sleep apnea syndrome patients. Chest 1999; 115:1519–24.

[27] Exar EN, Collop NA. The association of upper airway resistance with periodic limb movements. Sleep 2001;24(2):188–92.

[28] Guerrero M, Lepler L, Kristo D. The upper airway resistance syndrome masquerading as nocturnal asthma and successfully treated with an oral appliance. Sleep Breath 2001;5:93–5.

[29] Watanabe T, Mikami A, Taniguchi M, et al. Clinical characteristics of upper airway resistance syndrome. Psychiatry Clin Neurosci 1999;53: 331–3.

[30] Yoshida K. Oral device therapy for the upper airway resistance syndrome patient. J Prosthet Dent 2002;87(4):427–30.

[31] Pepin J, Veale D, Mayer P, et al. Critical analysis of the results of surgery in the treatment of snoring, upper airway resistance syndrome, and obstructive sleep apnea. Sleep 1996;19(9): S90–100.

[32] Krespi YP, Keidar A, Khosh MM, et al. The efficacy of laser-assisted uvulopalatoplasty in the management of obstructive sleep apnea and upper airway resistance syndrome. Operative Techniques in Otolaryngology—Head and Neck Surgery 1994; 5:235–43.

[33] Newman JP, Clerk AA, Moore M, et al. Recognition and surgical management of the upper airway resistance syndrome. Laryngoscope 1996; 106:1089–93.

[34] Lofaso F, Goldenberg F, Thebault C, et al. Effect of zopiclone on sleep, night-time ventilation and daytime vigilance in upper airway resistance syndrome. Eur Respir J 1997;10: 2573–7.

[35] Guilleminault C, Chervin R, Palombini L, et al. Radiofrequency (pacing and thermic effects) in the treatment of sleep-disordered breathing. Sleep 2000;23(S4):S182–6.

[36] Guilleminault C, Stoohs R, Shiomi T, et al. Upper airway resistance syndrome, nocturnal blood pressure monitoring, and borderline hypertension. Chest 1996;109(4):901–8.

[37] Guilleminault C, Kirisoglu C, Poyares D, et al. Upper airway resistance syndrome: a long-term outcome study. J Psychiatr Res 2006;40: 273–9.

SLEEP
MEDICINE
CLINICS

Sleep Med Clin 1 (2006) 483–489

Cyclic Alternating Pattern (CAP), Sleep Disordered Breathing, and Automatic Analysis

Christian Guilleminault, MD, BioID*, Agostinho da Rosa, PhD,
Chad C. Hagen, MD, Olga Prilipko, MD

A translational research using cyclic alternating pattern (CAP) analysis was performed in premenopausal women with complaints of fatigue and a low but abnormal apnea–hypopnea index (AHI). Results indicated that apnea and hypopnea do not describe well abnormal breathing during sleep in premenopausal women. Also, nonrapid eye movement (NREM) sleep scoring of CAP with automatic analysis was closely related to those obtained by two independent and blind to condition visual scorers. Pearson correlation coefficient showed a significant positive correlation between a visual analog fatigue scale score and CAP rate (scored either by automatic analysis or visual analysis). But no significant correlation was noted between visually scored EEG arousal and same scale. CAP is an important adjunction in the investigation of the sleep disturbance presented by sleep-disordered breathing (SDB) patients. The CAP automatic scoring system tested is sufficiently accurate to help CAP scoring. Current respiratory scoring criteria to evaluate severity of SDB in premenopausal women may be inadequate.

Introduction

Sleep disruption defined by changes in sleep stages scored according to the international criteria of Rechtschaffen and Kales [1] has correlated poorly with common complaints such as fatigue and decrements in alertness. The American Sleep Disorders Association (ASDA) addition of scoring EEG arousals of 3 seconds or longer [2] has improved the detection of sleep disruption but remains insensitive to more subtle EEG changes. Correlating sleep disruptions with subjective complaints is complicated by the occurrence of patients with a high AHI in the absence of excessive sleepiness complaints. This finding may be related to the fact that breathing events may terminate with a brainstem activation and not with an EEG arousal. Conversely, patients may also complain of tiredness and fatigue or cognitive impairment during the daytime while demonstrating a low number of EEG arousals, that again, fails to correlate with the severity of the daytime symptoms.

Stanford University Sleep Medicine Program, 401 Quarry Road, Stanford, CA 94305, USA
* Corresponding author.
E-mail address: cguil@stanford.edu (C. Guilleminault).

doi:10.1016/j.jsmc.2006.10.001
sleep.theclinics.com

Visual EEG sleep analysis by current scoring approaches may fail to adequately reflect the disturbances associated with SDB, thereby contributing to these discrepancies. Analysis of the CAP during nocturnal sleep has been used as a more sensitive investigation of sleep fragmentation in sleep disorders [3–6]. We report here on the development and validation of CAP scoring, and present a translational research application of CAP analysis to a case–control series of sleep-complaining women with mild Obstructive Sleep Apnea (OSA).

What Is Cyclic Alternating Pattern?

CAP is formed by electrocortical events that recur at regular intervals in the range of seconds during NREM sleep. These cortical events have been seen during the transition between sleep onset and establishment of consolidated delta sleep or spindle sleep during NREM sleep segments. These events are clearly distinguishable from the background EEG rhythms and identified by abrupt frequency shifts or amplitude changes [7–9] . Two adjacent phases (A and B) form a CAP cycle and recur within 2 to 60 seconds. When neither of the two phases is identifiable, sleep has reached a new stable state. Phase A is identified by transient events typically observed in NREM sleep. It includes EEG patterns of predominantly higher voltage and slower frequency, with a simultaneous faster frequency lower voltage in the background EEG. This increase in amplitude represents an activation phase that by definition is at least one third higher than the background EEG and lasts 2 to 60 seconds. Phase B follows phase A. It is the interval between two A phases, has a duration of 2 to 58 seconds, and has been defined by decreased EEG amplitude with EEG evidence of stages 1 to 2 NREM sleep.

Phase A has been subdivided into three subtypes [8]: subtype A1 is marked by a predominance of synchronized EEG activity with less than 20% desynchronized EEG activity (fast frequency and low amplitude). This appears as waveforms such as delta bursts, K-complex sequences, vertex waves, and polyphasic bursts of slow and fast EEG rhythms. Subtype A2 is scored in the presence of 20 to 50% desynchronized EEG activity with a predominance of polyphasic bursts. Subtype A3 is scored when at least 50% of the EEG activity is comprised of low amplitude fast rhythms such as K-alpha complexes, ASDA defined arousals [2], and polyphasic bursts.

The Development of Cyclic Alternating Pattern Scoring

More than 40 years ago "trace alternant" was defined in NREM sleep of infants in France. Since then, extensive research on cyclic EEG patterns occurring during NREM sleep in children and adults has produced broadening clinical applications. Much of the seminal work was performed in Italy over the past 20 years. The definition of CAP and different components was the result of pioneering work performed by the Parma University sleep laboratory, with investigation in normal subjects and in patients with sleep pathology [3,4,7–18].

The proposed definitions of CAP were originally based on visual scoring of EEG involving simultaneous analysis of at least four differently located EEG leads, one of which must be a central lead. The proposed definitions were reviewed and tested by a "CAP consensus workgroup" lead by Dr. Terzano, that met several times at the University of Parma. Early results of the workgroup included publication of the Atlas, rules, and recording techniques for the scoring of cyclic alternating pattern in human sleep that outlined how to visually score CAP and present results [8].

The CAP consensus group recognized early that the different EEG patterns analyzed when scoring CAP could easily be identified and quantified with computerized analysis. The development of automated computerized CAP scoring had obvious advantages for both research and clinical applications. Consistent with the clinical practice of scoring sleep and wake stages on a single a central EEG lead, automated scoring has also been based on data from a single central lead. The biomedical engineering laboratory of the University of Lisbon in Portugal, lead by Dr. Agostinho da Rosa, a member of the CAP consensus workgroup, initiated the pursuit of an automated CAP scoring method. Several segments of the project were portions of Masters or PhD theses. A continuous interaction between the Lisbon and Parma academic laboratories lead to the development of an analytic computerized system. Publications on reliability between automatic CAP scoring systems and arousal and CAP phase A [12,19–26] were published, using different tracings and segments from different parts of the night.

This analytic system was tested for accuracy in Europe, then financed in part by a sleep system company that permitted integration into a sleep scoring program. This "user-friendly" product was tested at two sites not involved in the development of the program (Federal University of Sao Paolo and Stanford University). Once tested and modified, the product was presented to members of the "CAP consensus workgroup" at a working meeting lasting several days. The workgroup reviewed sleep recordings from normal subjects and patients with data collected in European Data Format (EDF) [27] from different commercially available sleep systems. Short segments of polysomnograms with an EEG sampling frequency of 128Hz and C3/A2, C4/A1, Fp1–Fp2, and O1–O2 leads were presented to the panel of experts with request to indicate presence or absence of CAP. If CAP was judged present, the exact beginning and end of phase A and B were placed by one of the experts until the CAP sequence was over. This analysis was then presented to the panel of experts and reconsideration of scoring and rationale for changes were written down. Once consensus from experts was obtained, spectral analysis with relative and absolute EEG power calculated per 1-second window was displayed below each identified CAP phase for each EEG segment. The automated system's scoring was displayed on a third channel to allow visual inspection of agreement between the automated scoring system and the visual scoring of the expert consensus.

The experts reviewed the consensus and automated data evaluating discrepancies between the different methods. Some findings were expected. The human eye is poor at recognizing low alpha frequencies in the absence of associated mixtures of alpha and beta frequencies. Visual scoring also failed to recognize short bursts of low alpha power lasting up to 2 seconds. Additionally, visual scoring was not as sensitive as automated scoring for recognizing significant delta power of up to 50% in the presence of beta surges of up to 20% of the total reliable power for 1 or 2 seconds. This is particularly relevant, as it hinders the visual recognition of phase A or phase A1 termination. A discrepancy between the human eye and automated systems' recognition of subtle mid-line crossing and wave amplitude was also shown. Due to these discrepancies the computer interpreted the high amplitude segments to last longer than visual scorers did. This was a systematic discrepancy. As CAP is based on visual scoring, the consensus workgroup made a specific modification to the automated system's rule for ending phase A1 more consistent with the human eye's recognition of EEG amplitude and visual scoring. These default parameters were implemented at the first meeting day of the analytic program. Further investigation indicated much better agreement between experts and automated scoring after the modification.

Although the number of CAP cycles was in agreement between automated and expert scorers, interexpert scorer and expert-automated system disagreement related to duration of some CAP phases remained. These discrepancies were again related to the discriminative capabilities of the human eye, as shown by simultaneous EEG power analysis of the considered EEG segment. This human–computer scoring confrontation indicated, not surprisingly, that computer scoring was much more

consistent over time. It also showed that automated scoring was better at overall recognition of mean EEG frequencies during 1 second than the eye. Throughout the confrontation, at least one expert scorer scored as the computer did for each considered segment. Of importance, while the addition of other EEG leads for expert scorer analysis improved their interscorer agreement, it did not affect the automated versus visual scoring agreement. Following this meeting, selected parameters for CAP and CAP phase scoring were communicated to the company programmers and were implemented in the Somnologica Science 3-3 CAP automated analysis program.

Subsequent Validation of Automated Versus Visual Scoring

Sixteen hours of single-channel EDF format recordings were obtained from four different laboratories with either C4/A1 or C3/A2 channels and with different sampling frequencies (100, 128 or 256 Hz). Two 1-hour epochs of NREM sleep, one at the beginning of the night and one during the second half of the night, were extracted from each recording to obtain 16 files. The files were all scored by seven visual scorers, the proprietary system, and one automatic wavelet CAP-scoring system implemented on Matlab 6.0 [28].

Analysis of the agreement between the nine conditions was performed using an event-related analysis where an agreement is scored whenever two events have intersection longer than 0.5 seconds, which is designated as a "hit." This type of analysis allows identification of a "hit," "miss" (negative), or a "false positive" result. Comparing one scoring to another, this analysis can calculate the "sensitivity" of scoring A versus scoring B and the "positive predictive value." Likewise, scoring B is compared with scoring A and similar descriptive values obtained. If neither A nor B is considered as a reference, a "mutual agreement" (MA) score can be obtained. Additionally, a "number of disagreement" that includes false negative and false positives can be derived.

Using this approach, all nine scoring conditions were compared file by file (results of this analysis will be presented in a specific report; Rosa et al, personal communication). An interscorer sensitivity was calculated with one outlier scorer at 49.06, but all other scorers, the proprietary program, and the CAP-Lisbon automatic, oscillated between 72.36 and 84.69. The automated proprietary program obtained the highest interscorer sensitivity. The next highest sensitivity was a visual scorer from the University of Parma laboratory in which the visual CAP scoring system originated and the automated method was developed. The average mutual agreement oscillated between 60.35 and 73.82%, with again the highest score for the automated system, one outlier visual scorer, and the other scorers remaining around 70% to 71%. Investigation of the mutual agreement between all files visually scored by the most experienced and most knowledgeable CAP scoring laboratory had a mean percentage around 71%.

The results of this extensive process indicate that commercially available automatic algorithms can identify A phases (and therefore CAP cycle and CAP time) with precision that equals or exceeds that of traditional human scorers. It must be emphasized that this scoring was performed using only one EEG channel. Research protocols may have additional EEG channels, possibly improving scoring and agreement rates. Advantages of automated systems are their sensitivity to EEG changes and consistent scoring, which decreases variability when an analysis of a group of subjects (normal or patients) is performed. Even the most experienced scorers, as shown here, can have much larger scoring variability.

Translational research using CAP analysis in women with a complaint of "fatigue" and sleep disordered breathing

Methods

Patients

Participants were 40 women, age 18 to 38 years, referred to the Stanford Sleep Medicine Clinic with sleep-related complaints (see Table 1). All subjects were otherwise healthy and took no medications except for birth control pills.

Clinical evaluation of the upper airway indicated that 10 had tonsils >2 using Friedman and colleagues scales [29], and 27 had a Mallampati scale score of 3 or 4 [30]. Nasal evaluation indicated asymmetrical external nasal valve in 21, with presence of deviated septum in 20; enlarged inferior nasal turbinates in 29, and internal nasal valve collapse in 33. All presented evidence of narrow upper airway with a high and narrow hard palate in 29, and mandibular retroposition >2.2 mm in 13 [31]. Nasopharyngosopy demonstrated the presence of a small upper airway involving the base of the tongue in 18 subjects and nasopalatal impairment in 22 individuals.

Measures

All participants completed the Epworth Sleepiness Scale (ESS) and a visual analog scale (VAS) for daytime fatigue (ranging 0 for no fatigue to 100 mm, indicating "extreme fatigue to the point of not moving") [32]. The following variables were monitored during nocturnal polysomnography: four EEG leads (C3/A2, C4/A1, Fp3–Fp4, O1–O2), two electrooculograms, chin and leg EMGs, one ECG lead (modified V2 derivation), nasal cannula pressure transducer, mouth thermistor, neck microphone, chest and abdominal piezzoelectric bands, finger pulse-oxymetry, transcutaneous CO_2 electrode, and a position sensor. Lights out was determined by the subjects usual bedtime. A minimum of 7.5 hours of bedtime was requested.

Control Subjects

Twenty women, age 20 to 40 years (mean 29 = /±6 years) were recruited from the community. None

Table 1: Patients and control subjects clinical presentation

Variables	Patient group (n = 40)	Controls (n = 20)
Complaints		
Daytime fatigue	12	—
Sleep maintenance insomnia	18	—
Sleep onset insomnia	10	—
Ethnicity		
Caucasian	22	9
Far East Asian	12	8
South India	9	1
African American	2	1
Hispanic	1	1
Mean BMI (kg/m^2)	22.4 ± 1.1	23 ± 1.1
Past medical history		
Past adenotonsillectomy	18	4
Past orthodontic treatment	28	5
Wisdom teeth extraction early in life	22	—
Bruxism	17	—
Childhood asthma	5	—
Nasal allergies	25	—

reported health or sleep problems, and all were considered in good health with the absence of chronic medication intake except birth control pills. All had a clinical examination (see Table 1). None had wisdom teeth extraction, and all had an upper airway scored as normal size on physical evaluation. One subject had nasal septum deviation. They all completed the ESS and the VAS scales. Subjects underwent nocturnal polysomnography with monitoring of same variables and following the same protocol as patients.

Analysis

Recordings were scored for sleep and wake using international criteria. Abnormal breathing was scored using the definitions for apnea and hypopnea. As the nasal cannula pressure transducer was used, hypopnea was defined as a decrease of nasal flow by 30% of prior normal recording. An associated decrease in SaO_2 of 3% or an EEG arousal was required to score hypopneas. "Flow limitation" was scored based on nasal cannula pressure transducer indicating abnormal breathing characterized by a decrease of basal flow by 3% to 30% of prior normal breathing associated with a specific pattern of the nasal flow curve ("flattening" or "abrupt drop" at the beginning of inspiration) [33]. Four successive breaths with the pattern were needed to score a "flow limitation event." Also, 30-second epochs with tachypnea (defined as respiratory rate >20 breaths per minute during 30 seconds) were noted. The addition of "flow limitation" to AHI yielded the "respiratory disturbance index" (RDI). The lowest oxygen saturation (SaO_2) during the night and the number of 30-second epochs with snoring events were also tabulated.

All NREM sleep periods for both patients and control subjects were transformed to EDF format and transferred to a CD ROM. Each CD ROM was numbered to permit blinding of the scorers then analyzed for CAP. Two separate investigators performed the analysis. The CAP analysis was first performed based on C3/A2 or C4/A1 EEG lead, with selection of the lead based on the investigator's choice after inspecting the tracings. The analysis was also performed using the Somnologica Science 3.3 automated program. Then each recording was analyzed visually by the investigators using the four EEG leads available. Changes in the computer analysis could be done at this stage, and each investigator change was marked.

Comparison of results between controls and patients was performed using the Mann-Whitney test ($P = 0.05$ for significance). Correlation between CAP parameters and clinical variables were performed using Pearson correlation test. Percentages were analyzed by chi-square statistics.

Results

There were 40 patients and 20 controls. The mean age of patients was 28.6 ± 6 years and 27.9 ± 7 for controls (ns). The mean ESS score was 5 ± 2 and 4.5 ± 2 for patients and controls respectively (ns). All patients presented complaints of fatigue, and the mean VAS score for fatigue was 58 ± 10 for patients and 16 ± 5 for controls ($P = 0.0001$). Polysomnnography indicated that both groups had a relatively low AHI of 9 ± 3 and 1.1 ± 0.6 for patients and controls, respectively. Usage of RDI indicated a score of 22 ± 5 for patients and 1.5 ± 0.7 for controls. Both AHI and RDI were significantly different ($P = 0.0001$) between the groups. The mean lowest SaO_2 was $92 \pm 2.5\%$ for patients and $97 \pm 1\%$ for controls (chi-square statistics, $P = 0.001$). Analysis of EEG arousals 3 seconds or longer indicated a mean arousal index of 14 ± 3.1 for patients and 8.9 ± 4.6 for controls ($P = 0.001$).

The CAP rate percent was 59 ± 10 for patients versus 32 ± 5 for controls ($P = 0.01$). The mean CAP time in seconds for patients versus controls was 190 ± 37 and 73 ± 26 ($P = 0.01$), respectively. There was a mean of 382 ± 104 (patients) versus 135 ± 75 (controls) CAP cycles ($P = 0.01$).

These numbers were derived from comparison of the scores given by the two independent scorers. For patients, the CAP scores from automated and visual scoring were very close, with the mean difference of 0.3 for CAP rate and 1.1 for CAP cycle. Interestingly, the automatic scoring mean was between the mean for each of the two visual scorers.

Phase A1 in patients was calculated as 57 ± 14 by automatic scoring, 56 ± 15 by scorer A, and 59 ± 12 by scorer B. After conjoint review it was concluded to be at 57.8 ± 13.6. Phase A2 was calculated at 26 ± 10 by automatic analysis, 21 ± 11 by scorer A, and 27.6 ± 11 by scorer B. Opposing this trend, phase A3 was calculated at 15.3 ± 7 by automatic analysis, 19.8 ± 10 by scorer A and 14.3 ± 9 by scorer B.

For controls, there was a greater discrepancy. Mean CAP rate percent was still between that for the two visual scorers, but was 34 ± 7 for one scorer and 31 ± 6 for the other scorer, while automatic scoring yielded 31.9 ± 8. The presented score is the result of the review performed jointly by the two investigators to reconcile discrepancies. The initial scoring of the two investigators showed a large variation between the amount of phase A2 and A3. There were fewer discrepancies between scorers for controls after joint scoring index of phase A2 was scored at 25.8 ± 11.5 and index of phase A3 at 15.7 ± 7.5. The percentage of CAP phase A1 was 68.3 ± 17 with automatic analysis, 69 ± 18 for scorer A, and 68 ± 16 for scorer B. Percentage of CAP phase A2 was 19.5 ± 13 for automatic analysis, 20 ± 14 for scorer A, and 19 ± 12.6 for scorer B. Percentage of CAP phase A3 was 10.5 ± 7 for automatic scoring, 10 ± 6.5 for scorer A, and 10.9 ± 7.7 for scorer B.

Pearson correlation coefficient indicated a positive correlation ($r = 0.59$, $P = 0.0001$) between CAP rate and fatigue VAS score, while usage of arousal index did not reach significance.

Comments

Our study shows that young women with a low AHI present a remarkably higher RDI when attention is paid to less obvious breathing abnormalities than the AHI. This is an important finding, as many women may not be appropriately identified and treated if these more subtle respiratory abnormalities are not taken into consideration. Sleepiness was not the major complaint among the patient group, and the low, equivalent ESS scores between groups demonstrate this well, whereas "fatigue" was the primary feature. In practice, it is often difficult to articulate the nuances of fatigue and sleepiness with patients; however in our group, subjects clearly dissociated the "sleepiness" assessed with ESS from what they scored as "fatigue" using the VAS.

Our study demonstrates an important correlation between the CAP rate and the fatigue VAS score. The CAP rate was clearly different for patients compared with controls. The arousal index was also significantly different, but much less than the CAP rate. Clearly, the CAP rate allows investigation of changes in sleep architecture that are adequately detected with tabulation of short EEG arousals. There is an overlap between these EEG arousals and phase A3 of CAP, but there is no equivalent to the scoring of phase A2 of CAP to indicate a change in sleep architecture. Further work is needed to better understand what physiologic changes occur when such patterns are seen, but they clearly indicate a change from normal sleep architecture when present in large amounts.

Accurate quantification of CAP is dependent on sensitive recognition of these patterns. The definition of phase A2 and A3 call upon recognition of EEG frequency changes and determination of dominant EEG frequencies. This is a difficult task for the human eye. Training may improve results, but there will always be interrater discrepancies. The superior consistency of automated CAP scoring suggests that computers may arguably provide better CAP scoring than humans. However, the rules forming the basis of the automated programs are critical, and human scorers must always be able to overrule the computerized score. Efforts have been made over several years to develop and validate an automated scoring program. Usage of this automatic program has highlighted the difficulty in visually scoring CAP phase A2 and A3 even when using multiple EEG leads. It has also shown that an automatic CAP scoring program provides valid information on sleep architecture, and can be helpful when investigating sleep in normal and pathological conditions.

Acknowledgments

The Somnologica Science 3.3 program was the product of combined efforts from the bioengineering department, University of Lisbon (Portugal) and Flaga-Embla research and development team (Reykjavik, Iceland). It is currently the property of Medicare Inc (USA). The CAP consensus group was created by MG Terzano, MD, and involved the following individuals: R.D. Chevrin, S. Chokroverty, B. Consens, R. Ferri, C. Guilleminault, M.Hirshkovitz, Y.S. Huang, M.C. Lopes, M. Mahowald, H. Moldosky, L. Parrino, T. Roerhs, A. Rosa, R. Thomas, M. Zucconi, and A. Walters. The validation of the CAP automatic analysis program was performed without any commercial financial support. The Parma and Stanford meetings of the CAP consensus group members were supported by an educational unrestricted grant from Sanofi-Avantis.

References

[1] Rechtschaffen A, Kales A. Manual of standardized terminology: techniques and scoring system for sleep stages of human subjects. Los Angeles (CA): UCLA Brain Information Service/Brain Research Institute; 1968.

[2] American Sleep Disorders Association. EEG arousals: scoring rules and examples. A preliminary report from Sleep Disorders Atlas Task Force of the American Sleep Disorder Association. Sleep 1992;15:173–84.

[3] Terzano MG, Mancia D, Salati MR, et al. The cyclic alternating pattern as a physiologic component of normal NREM sleep. Sleep 1985;8:137–45.

[4] Terzano MG, Parrino L. Clinical applications of cyclic alternating pattern. Physiol Behav 1993; 54:807–13.

[5] De Gennaro L, Ferrara M, Spadini V, et al. The cyclic alternating pattern decreases as a consequence of total sleep deprivation and correlates with EEG arousals. Neuropsychobiology 2002;45:95–8.

[6] Zucconi M, Oldani A, Ferini-Strambi L, et al. Arousal fluctuations in non-rapid eye movement parasomnias: the role of cyclic alternating pattern as a measure of sleep instability. J Clin Neurophysiol 1995;12:147–54.

[7] Terzano MG, Parrino L, Spaggiari MC. The cyclic alternating pattern sequences in the dynamic organization of sleep. Electroencephalogr Clin Neurophysiol 1988;69:437–47.

[8] Terzano M, Parrino L, Smerieri A, et al. Atlas, rules, and recording techniques for the scoring of cyclic alternating pattern (CAP) in human sleep. Sleep Med 2002;3:187–99.

[9] Ferrillo F, Gabarra M, Nobili L, et al. Comparison between visual scoring of cyclic alternating pattern (CAP) and computerized assessment of slow EEG oscillations in the transition from light to deep non-REM sleep. J Clin Neurophysiol 1997;14:210–6.

[10] Parrino L, Boselli M, Spaggiari MC, et al. Cyclic alternating pattern (CAP) in normal sleep: poly-somnographic parameters in different age groups. Electroencephalogr Clin Neurophysiol 1998;107: 439–50.

[11] Terzano MG, Parrino L, Boselli M, et al. Polysom-nographic analysis of arousal responses in OSAS by means of the cyclic alternating pattern (CAP). J Clin Neurophysiol 1996;13:145–55.

[12] Rosa AC, Parrino L, Terzano M. Automatic detec-tion of cyclic alternating pattern (CAP) sequences in sleep: preliminary results. Electroencephalogr Clin Neurophysiol 1999;110:585–92.

[13] Ferri R, Parrino L, Smerieri A, et al. Cyclic alter-nating pattern and spectral analysis of heart rate variability during normal sleep. J Sleep Res 2000;9:13–8.

[14] Terzano MG, Parrino L, Rosa A, et al. CAP and arousals in the structural development of sleep: an integrative perspective. Sleep Med 2002;3: 221–2.

[15] Ferri R, Parrino L, Smerieri A, et al. Non-linear EEG measures during sleep: effects of the differ-ent sleep stages and Cyclic Alternating Pattern. Int J Psychophysiol 2002;43:273–86.

[16] Ferri R, Rundo F, Bruni O, et al. Dynamics of the EEG slow-wave synchronization during sleep. Clin Neurophysiol 2005;116:2783–95.

[17] Ferri R, Bruni O, Miano S, et al. All-night EEG power spectral analysis of the Cyclic Alternating Pattern components in young adult subjects. Clin Neurophysiol 2005;116:2429–40.

[18] Bruni O, Ferri R, Miano S, et al. Sleep cyclic alter-nating pattern in normal preschool-age children. Sleep 2005;28:220–30.

[19] Rosa AC, Allen Lima J. Fuzzy classification of microstructural dynamics of human sleep. Proc. 1996 IEEE Int. Conf. on Systems, Man and Cybernetics – Information, Intelligence and Systems, SMC'96 1996. Vol. 2, p. 1108–13.

[20] Allen Lima J, Rosa AC. Maximum likelihood based classification for the microstructure of human sleep. ACM SigBio Newslett 1997;17(3).

[21] Navona C, Barcaro U, Bonanni E, et al. An auto-matic method for the recognition and classifica-tion of the A-phases of the cyclic alternating pattern. Clin Neurophysiol 2002;113:1826–31.

[22] Largo R, Rosa A. Wavelets based detection of a phases in sleep EEG. Proc. II Int. Conf. Com-putacional Bioengineering. IST Press; 2005. Vol. 2, p. 1105–15.

[23] Largo R, Munteanu C, Rosa A. CAP event detection by wavelet and ga tuning. Proc. of IEEE- WISP Evolutionary Computation; 2005. CDRom.

[24] Ferri R, Bruni O, Miano S, et al. Inter-rater reli-ability of sleep cyclic alternating pattern (CAP) scoring and validation of a new computer -assis-ted CAP scoring method. Clin Neurophysiol 2005;116:696–707.

[25] Ferri R, Rundo F, Bruni O, et al. Regional scalp EEG slow-wave synchronization during sleep Cyclic Alternating Pattern A1 subtypes. Neurosci Lett 2006;404:352–7.

[26] Ferri R, Bruni O, Miano S, et al. The time struc-ture of the sleep Cyclic Alternating Pattern. Sleep 2006;29:693–9.

[27] Kemp B, Varri A, Rosa A, et al. A simple format for exchange of digitized polygraphic recordings. Electroencephalogr Clin Neurophysiol 1992;82: 391–3.

[28] MatLab v6.0 from Matwork Inc. http://www.mathworks.com.

[29] Friedman M, Tanyeri H, La Rosa M, et al. Clinical predictors of obstructive sleep apnea. Laryngo-scope 1999;109:1901–7.

[30] Mallampatti SR, Gatt SP, Gugino LD, et al. A clin-ical sign to predict difficult tracheal intubation: a prospective study. Can Anaesth Soc J 1985;32: 429–34.

[31] Kolar JC, Salter EM. Craniofacial anthropometry. Practical measurement of the head and face for clinical, surgical and research use. Springfield (IL): Charles C. Thomas; 1997.

[32] Johns MW. A new method for measuring day-time sleepiness: the Epworth sleepiness scale. Sleep 1991;14:540–5.

[33] Ayap I, Norman RG, Krieger AC, et al. Non-inva-sive detection of respiratory effort- related arousals (RERAs) by a nasal cannula/pressure transducer system. Sleep 2000;23:763–71.

SLEEP
MEDICINE
CLINICS

Sleep Med Clin 1 (2006) 491–498

Sleep-Related Breathing Disorders and Sleepiness

Max Hirshkowitz, PhD, D ABSM[a,b,*], Heidemarie Gast, MD[a,c]

Repetitive episodes of upper airway obstruction during sleep producing airflow cessation (apnea) or reduction (hypopnea) characterizes obstructive sleep apnea (OSA). OSA produces sleepiness that in some cases is debilitating [1,2]. Continuous positive airway pressure (CPAP) reportedly improves sleep-related breathing and relieves self-reported sleepiness.

Several instruments have been devised to assess self-reported sleepiness. The most common are the Stanford Sleepiness Scale (SSS) and the Epworth Sleepiness Scale (ESS). The Profile of Mood States (POMS), although originally designed to assess mood, is also popular in sleep research [3,4]. POMS scales for vigor, confusion, fatigue, and, to a lesser extent, depression and anger are sensitive to sleepiness. The SSS was designed for momentary assessment of introspective sleepiness [5]. Individuals choose between seven statements to describe their current state. The choices range from "feeling active and vital, alert, wide awake" to "almost in reverie, sleep-onset soon, lost struggle to remain awake." By contrast, the ESS is a questionnaire in which individuals disclose their expectation of "dozing" in eight soporific situations [6]. Johns [6,7] validated ESS on 54 patients with sleep-related breathing disorders (before and after treatment with CPAP) and 104 medical student controls. Controls had a mean score of 7.6, whereas patient mean was 14.3, declining to normal (7.4) after treatment. ESS scores have also been found to increase as a function of severity of sleep-disordered breathing [8].

Currently used objective tests of sleepiness include the multiple sleep latency test (MSLT) and maintenance of wakefulness test (MWT). These tests use electroencephalographic (EEG) criteria to objectively evaluate different aspects of sleepiness. MSLT indexes how quickly a person can fall asleep during nap opportunities scheduled at 2-hour intervals across the day. Using a similar procedure, MWT quantifies an individual's ability to overcome sleepiness and remain awake. Previous research has

This material is based upon work supported in part by the Office of Research and Development (R&D) Medical Research Service, Department of Veteran Affairs (VA) & the Friedrich-Ebert Foundation.
[a] Baylor College of Medicine, 1 Baylor Plaza, Houston, TX 77030, USA
[b] Sleep Disorders & Research Center, Michael E. DeBakey Veterans Affairs Medical Center (111i), 2002 Holcombe Blvd., Houston, TX 77030, USA
[c] Department of Neurology, Universität Witten/Herdecke, Witten, Germany
* Corresponding author. Sleep Center (111i), 2002 Holcombe Blvd., Bldg. 100, Rm 6C344, Houston, TX 77030.
E-mail address: maxh@bcm.tmc.edu (M. Hirshkowitz).

doi:10.1016/j.jsmc.2006.09.002

examined CPAP-related MSLT improvements in patients with OSA [9–13]. However, to our knowledge, MWT response in patients with polysomnographically diagnosed moderate to severe OSA to standard laboratory and titrated CPAP has not been evaluated in a randomized trial using untreated controls, although a test referred to as the MWT was used in one study [14]. Standardized MWT uses EEG criteria to determine sleep onset; the findings presented by Jenkinson and colleagues [14] were based on correlated behavioral measures.

The purpose of this study was to assess CPAP-related changes in sleepiness using standard subjective (ESS) and objective (MWT) measures and standard polysomnographic methods in patients with OSA in a randomized, parallel-group, repeated-measures design. To determine if alertness improved in association with CPAP, both self-report and objective measures were used. In this study, we were specifically interested in short-term changes (1–2 weeks) and whether differential CPAP use was associated with changes in sleepiness.

Methods

Subjects

Subjects were 29 men, age 33 to 64 years with OSA (apnea plus hypopnea index greater than 10 episodes per hour of sleep) randomly assigned to either untreated (n = 12) or CPAP treated (n = 17) groups. Diagnosis and optimal CPAP level were determined with attended, laboratory, comprehensive polysomnography. Mean (±SD) age did not differ between untreated (52.1 ± 6.7 years) and treated (52.5 ± 8.0 years) subjects. Educational levels were also comparable (14.8 ± 2.0 versus 15.5 ± 2.2 years, for untreated and treated groups, respectively). Finally, group difference for body mass index (33 ± 5.6 for untreated versus 40 ± 6.8 for treated) was not statistically significant.

As part of standard clinical protocol, subjects were interviewed, had a physical examination, provided a health history, and completed a questionnaire battery. Patients were excluded if they had moderate or severe pulmonary disease; congestive heart failure (New York Heart Association category III, IV); learning disabilities; current neurological conditions; suspected thought disorder or severe Axis II psychiatric disorder; suspected thyroid dysfunction, or acromegaly; or any condition other than OSA known to affect consciousness or alertness. Patients were also excluded if they were taking benzodiazepines, neuroleptics, central nervous system depressants, or psychostimulants. Written informed consent was obtained in accordance with the institutional review board guidelines.

Procedures

Our standard clinical questionnaire battery includes the Sleep Disorders Questionnaire [15], Cornell Medical Index, SSS [5], ESS [6], Beck Depression Inventory [16], and the Profile of Mood States [17].

Each subject slept three nights in the laboratory. The first night (Nt. 1) was used to diagnose OSA and screen for comorbid sleep disorders. CPAP titration was performed on the second night (Nt. 2). Subjects were titrated regardless of group assignment (treated or untreated). The third night (Nt. 3) scheduled approximately 1 to 2 weeks later (varying slightly between subjects but not between groups) was used for follow-up. Each subject randomly assigned to the treated group was given a CPAP machine and instructed to use it every night. Untreated subjects did not use CPAP (except for the titration night) until after the follow-up study night (Nt. 3).

Subjects slept in electrically shielded, sound-attenuated, temperature-controlled, private bedrooms. Subjects reported to the laboratory approximately 1 hour before their scheduled bedtime to have monitoring devices attached by a trained polysomnographic technologist. Just before going to sleep, the subject completed presleep questionnaires. Overnight sleep studies were recorded according to standard practice using Grass Instruments computerized polysomnographic systems. Electroencephalogram, electro-oculograms (left and right eye), electromyogram (submental and anterior tibialis), electrocardiogram, airflow (at the mouth and nares), respiratory effort (thoracic and abdominal movements), and oxygen saturation (pulse oximetry ear probe) were recorded. In the morning, the monitoring devices were removed and subjects completed a postsleep questionnaire.

The night technologist performed CPAP titration on Nt. 2. Subjects were shown a 20-minute videotape about OSA and CPAP therapy before titration to help prepare and orient them to the use of CPAPs and its benefits. Before starting the sleep study, a nasal CPAP mask was fitted and applied with an initial pressure of 3 cm H_2O. After sleep onset, pressures were increased until apnea and hypopnea events were minimized. A board-certified sleep specialist determined optimal CPAP during record review. Each study subject in the treated group was provided a CPAP machine, was given further instructions on its use, and had an opportunity to ask questions. Additionally, we encouraged subjects to call immediately if there were any problems.

Recording and scoring technique followed currently published standards for human subjects; this included procedures for sleep stages [18], leg

Table 1: **Sleep parameters at baseline in patients with OSA**

	U (N = 12)		T (N = 17)		TC (N = 9)		TNC (N = 8)	
Variable	Mean	SD	Mean	SD	Mean	SD	Mean	SD
AI	21.6	19.8	23.5	26.2	36.3	30.4	9.0	7.3
AHI	39.7	25.6	45.5	32.1	60.1	34.3	29.0	20.7
Longest apnea (sec)	52.4	23.5	53.0	23.8	55.7	24.6	49.9	24.2
SaO$_2$ nadir (%)	78.0	14.7	69.5	20.4	64.3	17.5	75.3	23.0
PLM index	27.0	36.5	23.5	42.0	29.5	53.3	16.7	26.2
PLM arousal index	9.7	11.3	8.0	14.6	7.5	16.0	8.7	13.9

AI and AHI differed significantly between TNC and TC groups. No other group differences for any other variables were found.
Abbreviations: T, treated; TC, treated compliant; TNC, treated noncompliant; U, untreated.

movement [19], and respiration [20]. Obstructive respiratory events were differentiated as apneas (10-second or longer airflow cessation) or hypopneas (10-second or longer, 50% or more decline in airflow with desaturation, a termination arousal, or asynchronous breathing).

Maintenance of Wakefulness Tests (MWT) were performed on the day after the diagnostic sleep evaluation and the day after the follow-up sleep study [21]. We used a 20-minute version of MWT. MWT sessions were scheduled at 2-hour intervals commencing 2 hours after awakening from the previous night's sleep. During test sessions, electrophysiologic data required to detect sleep onset and score sleep stages were recorded. Recording montage included central and occipital electroencephalograms, left and right eye electro-oculograms, and submentalis electromyogram. Sleep rooms were darkened and quiet during testing. Subjects were tested in their street clothes and were not permitted to remain in bed between test sessions. Subjects were instructed to *attempt to remain awake* during the 20-minute test session. Finally, we also administered a neuropsychological test battery at baseline and follow-up (reported elsewhere).

Results

Data were analyzed using SAS statistical software. To test group comparability, *t* tests were used.

Sleepiness measures were analyzed using within-subjects general linear models (GLM) analysis of variance (ANOVA) procedures with main effects for group (treated [T] versus untreated [U]) and session (baseline versus follow-up). The interaction effect for group × session provided a test for the differential effect of CPAP on a given sleepiness measure. Additional GLM analyses were conducted with a trifurcated group factor (treated compliant [TC], treated noncompliant [TNC], and untreated [U]) to assess whether the amount of CPAP use affected outcome. Subjects using CPAP more than 5 hours per night (based on hour meter readings at follow-up) were classified as TC; other treated subjects were classified as TNC.

Group comparability testing

To determine group comparability, Apnea Index (AI), Apnea plus Hypopnea Index (AHI), the duration of the longest apnea episode, the SaO$_2$ nadir, periodic leg movement (PLM) index, and PLM arousal index were compared between groups at baseline. No significant group differences were found between treated (T) and untreated (U) subjects (Table 1). However, when CPAP use was considered, group differences emerged with significantly lower ($P < .05$) AI and AHI for subjects in the TNC group compared with those in the TC group.

Table 2: **SSS and ESS scores at baseline and follow-up in treated (n = 17) and untreated (n = 12) groups**

		Treated		Untreated		Group × session
	Session	Mean	SD	Mean	SD	P value
Stanford Sleepiness	Baseline	3.61	1.51	4.06	1.58	.154
Scale	Follow-up	2.82	1.81	4.00	1.53	
Epworth Sleepiness	Baseline	15.76	4.93	17.00	6.16	.006
Scale	Follow-up	8.59	4.39	15.83	5.39	

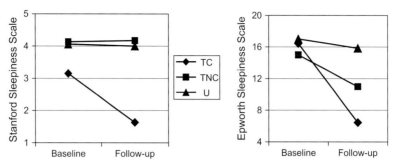

Fig. 1. SSS and ESS Scores for TC, TNC, and U groups at baseline and follow-up.

Self-reported sleepiness

Stanford Sleepiness Scale

Stanford Sleepiness Scale was administered at each MWT session. The mean SSS scores across the day were calculated for each subject. Table 2 displays SSS group (T and U) means at baseline and follow-up. Groups did not differ at baseline and the group × session interaction was not significant. There was a trend ($P = .078$) toward treated subjects having lower SSS scores at follow-up than untreated subjects.

Analyses were also conducted taking CPAP usage into account. The left panel of Fig. 1 illustrates SSS scores for each group (TC, TNC, and U) by session. A significant group × session interaction effect ($P = .015$) was found. SSS did not differ significantly between groups at baseline; however, statistically reliable SSS score decrement occurred in the TC group compared with the U group ($P < .001$) and the TNC group ($P < .001$).

Epworth Sleepiness Scale

Epworth Sleepiness Scale means at baseline and follow-up for treated and untreated subjects are also shown in Table 2. No significant group differences for ESS scores were seen at baseline. By contrast, a pronounced group × session interaction effect was found for ESS scores ($P = .006$) reflecting a large decrease in the T group compared with little change in the U group.

Continuous positive airway pressure usage differentially affected ESS scores. The right panel of Fig. 2 illustrates ESS scores for each group at baseline and follow-up. A robust group × session interaction was found ($P < .001$). Although no group differences were observed at baseline, at follow-up significant improvements were found in the TC group compared with the U group ($P < .001$) and the TNC group ($P = .027$). A near-significant improvement was also found in the TNC groups ($P = .051$) compared with the untreated group.

Profile of Mood States

Profile of Mood States subscale scores for vigor, fatigue, confusion, anger, tension, and depression at baseline and follow-up for T and UT are shown on Table 3. Significant group × session interactions were found for the vigor and fatigue scales. Fig. 2 illustrates mean POMS scores for each scale for TC, TNC, and U groups.

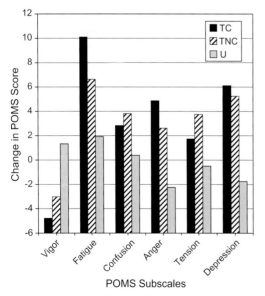

Fig. 2. Profile of mood state changes for TC, TNC, and U groups at baseline and follow-up.

Objectively assessed sleepiness

Each MWT session was scored for sleep latency using three different criteria. Simple sleep latency (SIMPL-SL) was defined as the elapsed time from lights out to the first epoch (1 epoch = 30 seconds) of any stage of sleep. Unequivocal sleep latency (UNEQV-SL) was defined as the elapsed time from lights out to the first three consequent epochs of stage 1 or any other stage, or one epoch of any other sleep stage. Finally, nonwake, nonstage one sleep latency (NWN1-SL) was defined as the elapsed time from lights out to the first epoch of

Table 3: **POMS subscale scores at baseline and follow-up for treated and untreated groups**

Subscale	Session	Treated Mean	SD	Untreated Mean	SD	Group × session P value
Vigor	Baseline	11.24	5.61	14.73	5.76	.047
	Follow-up	15.18	6.16	13.40	6.77	
Fatigue	Baseline	14.29	6.44	12.42	5.99	.017
	Follow-up	6.07	5.39	10.50	7.11	
Confusion	Baseline	4.93	6.69	1.83	2.72	.336
	Follow-up	1.65	3.89	1.44	3.54	
Anger	Baseline	9.63	11.24	5.75	5.05	.126
	Follow-up	5.88	8.06	8.00	4.57	
Tension	Baseline	4.47	5.59	1.91	3.42	.347
	Follow-up	1.75	5.45	2.40	5.25	
Depression	Baseline	13.29	15.28	4.75	3.74	.144
	Follow-up	7.59	9.06	6.50	5.60	

stage two, three, four, or REM sleep. Table 4 shows mean MWT sleep latencies at baseline and follow-up for treated and untreated subjects. GLM ANOVAs showed significant group × session interactions for all three sleep latency measures, notwithstanding latency equivalencies at baseline. Treated group mean sleep latencies increased by 3.89, 4.07, and 4.29 minutes for SIMPL-SL, UNEQ-UV-SL, and NWN1-SL, respectively. By contrast, in untreated patients, SIMPL-SL increased by only 0.66 minutes and decreased more than a minute on UNEQV-SL and NWN1-SL measures.

Analyses were also conducted taking CPAP usage into account. Fig. 3 illustrates MWT UNEQV-SL scores at baseline and follow-up for TC, TNC, and U groups. Statistical analysis found a significant group × session interaction effect (P = .001). At baseline, treated and untreated groups did not differ; however, there was a trend toward the TNC group having longer latencies (9.6 minutes) than the other groups (7.5 min for U [P = .28] and 6.3 for TC [P = .16]). Improvement at follow-up reached statistical significance when the untreated group was compared with either treated group (P = .035 for TC and P = .014 for TNC); however, TC and TNC groups were equivalent at follow-up

(P = .979). Fig. 3 also shows the percent of patients in each group with mean MWT latency ≥12 minutes at baseline and follow-up. Individual MWT sessions are illustrated in Fig. 4 for each group.

Discussion

The results of this study indicate significant CPAP-related improvements in objectively and subjectively measured sleepiness in patients with OSA. When CPAP use is considered, a more complex pattern of results emerges. On ESS there was a stepwise improvement, proceeding from no treatment, to partial CPAP use, to full use. The group that was fully compliant attained near-normal values for ESS within 2 weeks. Momentary assessment measures of sleepiness (SSS) were less sensitive to the presence of CPAP treatment but were more sensitive to amount of use. Interestingly, the pattern of changing sleepiness detected by ESS could also be observed in POMS vigor and fatigue scale scores. Thus, momentary assessment of sleepiness provides different information than composite global self-evaluation.

For objectively assessed sleepiness (using MWT), equivalent endpoints were attained by treated subjects who fully used CPAP therapy and by subjects

Table 4: **MWT latencies at baseline and follow-up in treated and untreated groups**

	Session	Treated Mean	SD	Untreated Mean	SD	Group × session P value
SIMPL-SL (minutes)	Baseline	6.43	4.76	5.95	3.04	.013
	Follow-up	10.32	5.67	5.29	2.11	
UNEQV-SL (minutes)	Baseline	7.85	4.75	7.47	3.13	.001
	Follow-up	11.92	5.82	6.44	3.31	
NWN1-SL (minutes)	Baseline	9.59	4.99	9.21	3.63	.003
	Follow-up	13.80	5.35	7.87	2.86	

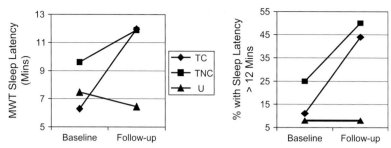

Fig. 3. Maintenance of wakefulness test sleep results for TC, TNC, and U groups at baseline and follow-up. The left panel shows mean unequivocal sleep latencies across test sessions, and the right panel shows the percentage of subjects with a mean latency ≥12 minutes.

who only partially complied with the treatment regimen. These two self-selected groups, however, differed at baseline both for condition severity (AI and AHI) and objective sleepiness (MWT latency). Thus, less sleepy patients (by MWT criteria) used CPAP less but achieved the same endpoint (mean MWT latency of approximately 12 minutes) as sleepier patients who used CPAP 5 hours (or more) per night. Interestingly, 12 minutes is the MWT latency representing the 95th percentile of normal, according to normative values published by Doghramji and colleagues [22]. It seems, therefore, that with 2 weeks of CPAP use, patients can improve to at least the low end of the normal range. Furthermore, it appears that some patients will use CPAP only enough to achieve this level of alertness. This finding concords with the well-documented long-term interrelationship between CPAP use and self-reported sleepiness; that is, patients who do not report sleepiness are more likely to abandon using CPAP [23].

Our findings replicate previous works illustrating improvement of self-reported sleepiness after CPAP therapy. It is notable that these improvements are discernable within a couple of weeks. Johns [6,7]

found an approximate 50% CPAP-related improvement from ESS baseline (14.3) to an endpoint within the normal range. In the current study we found comparable improvement (15.8 at baseline to 8.6 at endpoint with CPAP). However, this included both patients who used CPAP regularly and patients who did not. ESS improvement in compliant patients was more dramatic, reaching an endpoint mean of 6.4 after approximately 2 weeks. These CPAP-related improvement in ESS scores replicates other recent reports [12–14,24,25].

Studies examining objectively measured sleepiness commonly use the MSLT. Mixed results are reported in response to CPAP therapy. Lamphere and coworkers [9] reported a robust decline in MSLT-indexed sleepiness associated with CPAP therapy in the 39 patients they tested. Although there was no untreated control group, a 6-minute increase after 1 night and a 9.6-minute increase after 2 weeks of CPAP therapy were noted. By contrast, in a controlled study, Brown and colleagues [10] found a nonsignificant mean MSLT latency increase from 6.6 minutes at baseline to 7.6 minutes (SD 5.4) after 3 weeks of treatment in a group of 19 patients. Another study group [11] reported small but

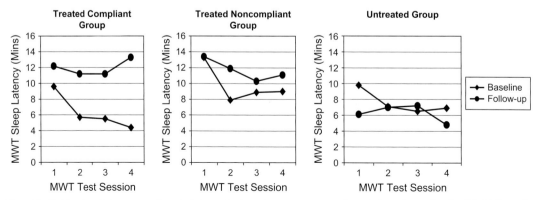

Fig. 4. Individual maintenance of wakefulness test session mean unequivocal sleep latencies for TC, TNC, and U groups at baseline and follow-up.

significant MSLT differences between CPAP-treated and conservatively treated patients when comparing baseline measures with 3-month follow-up measures. Using their nonstandard criteria for sleep onset (latency to a 20-second epoch of any sleep stage), an increase in mean latency of slightly more than 2 minutes was found for the CPAP-treated group, whereas the other group's mean declined approximately 1 minute. In a more recent study by the same group [12], MSLT latency declined from 7.2 to 6.1 minutes ($P < .05$). These mixed results concerning CPAP-related MSLT improvement may reflect variable use of the machine, comorbid disorders producing somnolence, or a continued high drive to sleep among some patients with OSA notwithstanding therapy.

MSLT differs from MWT in several ways; however, the critical manner in which these tests diverge relates to the instructions. MSLT instructs individuals "not to resist sleep," and thereby it provides what has become our best technique for assessing the physiological *drive to sleep*. MWT provides individuals with the opposite directive; that is, "resist sleep." In doing so, it does not seek to measure the *drive to sleep* but rather the alerting system's ability to overcome this drive. As such, we may consider MWT as an objective measure for "overwhelming sleepiness." In the current study, CPAP clearly improved the ability of patients with OSA to resist overwhelming sleepiness. Finally, it is intriguing that in the current study, patients appear to be titrating their CPAP usage to their level of overwhelming sleepiness.

References

[1] Guilleminault C, Partinen MD, Quera-Salva MA, et al. Determinants of daytime sleepiness in obstructive sleep apnea. Chest 1988;94:32–7.

[2] Flemons WW, Tsai W. Quality of life consequences of sleep-disordered breathing. J Allergy Clin Immunol 1997;99:750–6.

[3] Kribb NB, Pack AI, Kline LR, et al. Effects of one night without nasal CPAP treatment on sleep and sleepiness in patients with obstructive sleep apnea. Am Rev Respir Dis 1993;147:1162–8.

[4] Derderian SS, Bridenbaugh R, Rajagopal KR. Neuropsychologic symptoms in obstructive sleep apnea improve after treatment with nasal continuous positive airway pressure. Chest 1988;94:1023–7.

[5] Hoddes E, Zarcone V, Smythe H, et al. Quantification of sleepiness: a new approach. Psychophysiol 1973;10:431–6.

[6] Johns MW. A new method for measuring daytime sleepiness: the Epworth Sleepiness Scale. Sleep 1991;14:540–5.

[7] Johns MW. Reliability and factor analysis of the Epworth Sleepiness Scale. Sleep 1992;15:376–81.

[8] Hirshkowitz M, Gokcebay N, Iqbal S, et al. Epworth sleepiness scale and sleep-disordered breathing: replication and extension. Sleep Res 1995;24:249.

[9] Lamphere J, Roehrs T, Wittig R, et al. Recovery of alertness after CPAP in apnea. Chest 1989;96:1364–7.

[10] Brown WD, Jamieson AO, Becker PM, et al. Cognitive, emotional, and behavioral correlates of obstructive sleep apnea and the effects of continuous positive airway pressure (CPAP) treatment: the importance of a control group. Sleep Res 1991;20:213.

[11] Engleman HM, Cheshire KE, Deary IJ, et al. Daytime sleepiness, cognitive performance and mood after continuous positive airway pressure for the sleep apnoea/hypopnoea syndrome. Thorax 1993;48:911–4.

[12] Engleman HM, Martin SE, Deary IJ, et al. Effect of continuous positive airway pressure treatment on daytime function in sleep apnoea/hypopnoea syndrome. Lancet 1994;343:572–5.

[13] Engleman HM, Kingshott RN, Wraith PK, et al. Randomized placebo-controlled crossover trial of continuous positive airway pressure for mild sleep apnea/hypopnea syndrome. Am J Respir Crit Care Med 1999;159:461–7.

[14] Jenkinson C, Davies RJO, Mullins R, et al. Comparison of therapeutic and subtherapeutic nasal continuous positive airway pressure for obstructive sleep apnoea: a randomised prospective parallel trial. Lancet 1999;353:2100–5.

[15] Douglass AB, Bornstein R, Nino-Murcia G, et al. The sleep disorders questionnaire I: creation and multivariate structure of SDQ. Sleep 1994;17:160–7.

[16] Beck AT, Steer RA. Beck depression inventory manual. San Antonio TX: San Antonio Psychological Corporation; 1987.

[17] McNair DM, Lorr M, Droppleman LF. Manual of the profile of mood states. San Diego, CA: Educational and Industrial Testing Service; 1971.

[18] Rechtschaffen A, Kales A. A manual of standardized, techniques and scoring system for sleep stages in human subjects. Washington DC: NIH Publication No. 204, US Government Printing Office; 1968.

[19] ASDA Task Force. Bonnet M, Carley D, Guilleminault C, et al. Recording and scoring leg movements. Sleep 1993;16:748–59.

[20] Bornstein SK. Respiratory monitoring during sleep: polysomnography. In: Guilleminault C, editor. Sleeping and waking disorders: indications and techniques. Menlo Park, CA: Addison-Wesley; 1982. p. 183–212.

[21] Mitler MM, Gujavarty KS, Browman CP. Maintenance of wakefulness test: a polysomnographic technique for evaluating treatment efficacy in patients with excessive somnolence. EEG Clin Neurophysiol 1982;53:658–61.

[22] Doghramji K, Mitler MM, Sangal RB, et al. A normative study of the maintenance of wakefulness test (MWT). EEG Clin Neurophysiol 1997;103: 554–62.

[23] McArdle N, Devereux G, Heidarnejad H, et al. Long-term use of CPAP therapy for sleep apnea/hypopnea syndrome. Am J Respir Crit Care Med 1999;159:1108–14.

[24] Meurice JC, Marc I, Series F. Efficacy of auto-CPAP in the treatment of obstructive sleep apnea/hypopnea syndrome. Am J Respir Crit Care Med 1996;153:794–8.

[25] Redline S, Adams N, Strauss ME, et al. Improvement of mild sleep-disordered breathing with CPAP compared to conservative therapy. Am J Respir Crit Care Med 1998;157:858–65.

SLEEP
MEDICINE
CLINICS

Sleep Med Clin 1 (2006) 499–511

Sleep-Related Breathing Disorders and Continuous Positive Airway Pressure–Related Changes in Cognition

Heidemarie Gast, MD[a,c], Susanne Schwalen, MD[c],
Hubert Ringendahl, MD[c], Johannes Jörg, MD[c],
Max Hirshkowitz, PhD, D ABSM[a,b],*

Obstructive sleep apnea (OSA) is the most common sleep-related breathing disorder. It is characterized by repetitive episodes of upper airway obstruction during sleep, leading to markedly reduced (hypopnea) or absent (apnea) airflow. This condition usually is associated with loud snoring, hypoxemia, and excessive daytime sleepiness [1].

In addition to excessive sleepiness, the literature indicates that a variety of sequelae accompany OSA. These sequelae include paranoia and personality changes, impaired work efficiency, more frequent automobile accidents, reduced quality of life, and cognitive impairment [2–8].

The neuropsychologic deficits that reportedly occur in individuals who have OSA include perceptual-organizational, attention, vigilance, concentration, memory, general intellectual, and psychomotor impairments [9–15]. Results usually derive from cross-sectional studies, comparing untreated patients with a control group. For example, Lee and colleagues [16] compared 17 subjects who had OSA (an apnea plus hypopnea index [AHI] ranging from 12–85 events per hour of sleep) with 16 healthy controls. Groups were matched for age, ethnicity, gender, IQ, and years of education. Subjects were administered the Wisconsin Card Sorting Test (WCST), Trail Making Test (TMT) B, Wechsler Adult Intelligence Scale-Revised Digit Span (WAIS-R Digit Span) Test, a computerized version of the Tower Puzzle, a serial subtraction task, the Controlled

This article is based on work supported in part by the Office of Research and Development (R&D) Medical Research Service, Department of Veteran Affairs (VA) and the Friedrich-Ebert Foundation.
[a] Baylor College of Medicine, 1 Baylor Plaza, Houston, TX 77030, USA
[b] Sleep Disorders & Research Center, Michael E. DeBakey Veterans Affairs Medical Center (111i), 2002 Holcombe Blvd., Houston, TX 77030, USA
[c] Department of Neurology, Universität Witten/Herdecke, Witten, Germany
* Corresponding author. Sleep Center (111i), 2002 Holcombe Blvd., Bldg. 100, Rm 6C344, Houston, TX 77030.
E-mail address: maxh@bcm.tmc.edu (M. Hirshkowitz).

doi:10.1016/j.jsmc.2006.10.006

Oral Word Association from the Multilingual Aphasia Examination, the California Verbal Learning Test (CVLT) (trial 1), a Choice Reaction Time task, and the Park and Holzman's procedure. The OSA group showed significantly more perseveration errors on the WCST and tended to be less verbally fluent (ie, showed greater deficits in the retrieval of information from semantic memory) than normal controls.

Treatment intervention paradigms also have been used to investigate OSA-related cognitive impairments. Continuous positive airway pressure (CPAP) currently is the preferred treatment for OSA. It provides constant pressure to offset airway collapse, thereby maintaining airway patency. When pressure is properly titrated, sleep-disordered breathing events can be minimized.

Some studies report dramatically improved neuropsychologic functions after OSA is treated with CPAP [13,17]. By contrast, only modest or no improvements in neuropsychologic test scores are found when CPAP-treated groups are compared with untreated or placebo-treated groups [18–23]. Thus, results are inconsistent across studies, but these differences probably arise from differences in experimental design. Some studies test patients who are available in the clinical setting without a parallel group for comparison. In such designs, it is difficult to know to which factor(s) one should attribute treatment-related changes. Nonetheless one study with a randomized-group design reported significant CPAP-related improvements on a majority of neuropsychologic tests [24].

Factors playing a critical role in study results include practice effects, OSA severity, and CPAP use. Brown and colleagues [18] randomly assigned subjects who had AHIs of less than 20 into treated and untreated groups. They found large practice effects on neuropsychologic test scores; however, CPAP use was not reported. In another study reported in abstract form [21], OSA patients (AHI > 15) were randomly assigned to treated (optimal CPAP) and control (2 cm H_2O CPAP) groups. Improvements were found in both groups, but only one test (Digit Vigilance–Time) showed CPAP-related improvement beyond practice. CPAP use was not reported. As part of his dissertation project, Bailey [20] compared changes from baseline in treated and untreated subjects after 3 nights, finding improvement in only 1 (visual memory) of 18 neuropsychologic measures. In one study by Engleman and coworkers [22], patients who had mild OSA (AHI = 10) had CPAP-related improvement in the Digit Symbol Substitution Test and Paced Auditory Serial Addition Test (PASAT). A trend was also found for the TMT. CPAP usage was poor (mean, 2.8 hours per night), however. Engleman's [21] other study compared CPAP with conservative treatment (presumably weight loss) at baseline and at 3-month follow-up. CPAP use was good (mean, 5.9 hours per night), but no CPAP-related improvements were found on any psychomotor or cognitive test. Finally in the study by Mendelson and coworkers [19], treatment-related improvements were found for explicit memory, but AHI differed greatly between groups at baseline. By contrast, the results from 1700 patients tested with delayed word recall tests, WAIS-R Digit Symbol Substitution subtest, and the word fluency test showed no relationship between severity of sleep apnea (index by overnight respiratory disturbance index) and cognitive function [25].

The purpose of the authors' present study was to assess CPAP-related neuropsychologic changes in patients who had OSA using a randomized, parallel-group, within-subject design. This design allowed assessment of both CPAP-related changes and practice effects. To determine if cognitive changes occur in association with CPAP, a large battery of neuropsychologic tests was used. Test selection was guided by publications showing neuropsychologic impairment or dysfunction in patients who have OSA. This study specifically investigated in short-term changes (1–2 weeks) and the influence, if any, of CPAP use.

Methods

Subjects

Thirty-four men, age 33 to 64 years, who had OSA (AHI > 10 episodes per hour of sleep) served as subjects in the present study. Subjects were assigned randomly to one of two groups: 17 in the treated group, and 12 in the untreated group. Five subjects (two from the treated group and three from the untreated group) were excluded because of protocol violations. Table 1 shows the demographic data for subjects in each group. All subjects were evaluated at the Sleep Disorders and Research Center over an 8-month period.

Table 1: Subject demographics (mean ± SD)

Characteristic	Untreated	Treated
Age (years)	52.09 ± 6.67	52.5 ± 7.97
Education (years)	14.82 ± 1.99	15.47 ± 2.19
Weight (lbs)	245.8 ± 26.45	267.6 ± 34.21
Height (inches)	73 ± 8.5	69 ± 3.8
Body mass Index	33 ± 5.6	40 ± 6.8

As part of standard clinical protocol, subjects were interviewed, had a physical examination, provided a health history, and completed a questionnaire battery. Additionally, an inventory of current medications was obtained. Patients aged 30 to 65 years with hallmark symptoms of sleep apnea were referred for additional screening. Patients were excluded if they moderate or severe pulmonary disease, congestive heart failure (New York Heart Association category III or IV), learning disabilities, current major psychiatric illness, current neurologic disease (eg, dementia, recent head trauma, stroke, narcolepsy, multiple sclerosis, or amyotrophic lateral sclerosis), suspected thyroid dysfunction, acromegaly, or other conditions affecting consciousness or alertness other than OSA. Patients also were excluded if they were taking benzodiazepines, neuroleptics, central nervous system depressants, or psychostimulants. If a thought disorder or severe Axis II psychiatric disorder was suspected, the patient was excluded from the study. Patients suffering from mild-to-moderate Axis I disorders were not excluded because these disorders are common among patients who have OSA [26,27]. Written informed consent was obtained in accordance with the institutional review board guidelines.

Procedure

The questionnaire battery included the Sleep Disorders Questionnaire [28], the Cornell Medical Index, the Stanford Sleepiness Scale, the Epworth Sleepiness Scale, the Beck Depression Inventory, and the Profile of Mood States.

Subjects who met selection criteria and agreed to participate were scheduled for daytime neuropsychologic testing and Maintenance of Wakefulness Test (MWT) on the day following their regularly scheduled diagnostic sleep evaluation at the Sleep Disorders and Research Center. All subjects were asked to not drink any caffeinated beverages after 5 PM on the first, second, and third night of polysomnography and during all days of testing.

Subjects slept a minimum of 3 nights in the laboratory. Night 1 was to quantify sleep-disordered breathing and screen for comorbid sleep disorders. Night 2 was for nasal CPAP titration. Titration proceeded according to standard clinical protocol. Patients were titrated regardless of group assignment (as treated or untreated). Night 3 was scheduled at least 1 week after night 1 (varying slightly among subjects but not between groups). Subjects in the treated group slept using CPAP every night during the interim between night 2 and night 3 (inclusive). The untreated group did not receive CPAP (except for the titration night) until after night 3.

Polysomnography

Subjects slept in private, electrically shielded, sound-attenuated, temperature-controlled bedrooms. Subjects reported to the laboratory approximately 1 hour before scheduled bedtime to complete pre-sleep questionnaires and have monitoring devices attached by a trained polysomnography technician. Full-night sleep studies were recorded according to standard practice using Grass Heritage computerized polysomnographic systems (Grass Instruments, Quincy, Massachusetts). Surface electrodes were used to record electroencephalographic, electro-oculographic, electromyographic (submental and anterior tibialis), and ECG activities. Nasal-oral thermocouples monitored airflow; thoracic and abdominal movements indicated respiratory effort. The respiratory tracings were scored for the presence of apneas ($\geq$ 10-second cessation in nasal-oral airflow) or hypopneas ($\geq$ 10-second reduction of nasal-oral airflow of $\geq$ 50%). Blood oxygen saturation (SaO_2) was monitored with pulse oximetry (with the sensor placed on the earlobe). All polysomnographic procedures were noninvasive. Recording and scoring techniques, including procedures for sleep stages [29], respiration [30], and leg movement [31], followed currently published standards for human subjects. In the morning, the monitoring devices were removed, and the subjects completed a postsleep questionnaire detailing subjective sleep quality and quantity.

Continuous positive airway pressure titration

During night 2 CPAP was titrated. Before titration, subjects were shown a 20-minute videotape about OSA and CPAP therapy. The video helps prepare and orient patients to CPAP use and its benefits. Before the sleep study was started, a nasal CPAP mask was fitted and applied. Initial pressure was approximately 3 cm H_2O. After sleep onset, the technician gradually increased the pressure until apnea and hypopnea events were minimized. A board-certified sleep specialist reviewed the records to determine that optimal CPAP pressure and CPAP machines were provided to study subjects. When patients received the CPAP machine, they were given further instructions on its use and had the opportunity to ask questions. Patients also were encouraged to call immediately if any problems arose.

Neuropsychologic assessment

All testing was administered and scored by the author (HG) using standardized procedures and instructions. Subjects received two identical neuropsychologic evaluations on two occasions. Tests were presented in the same order for all subjects (see Table 2). Each neuropsychologic

Table 2: Neuropsychologic tests and presentation order within sessions

Test Battery Session	Test Name	Abbreviation
1	Mini Mental Status Examination	MMSE[a]
	California Verbal Learning Test	CVTL
	Modified Wisconsin Card-sorting Test	WCST
2	Paced Auditory Serial Addition Task	PASAT
	Bedside Assessment of Executive Cognitive Impairment-Executive Interview	EXIT
3	Tower of Toronto	TOT 3 and 4
	Stroop Color-Word Test	Stroop
	Wechsler Adult Intelligence Scale – revised Digit Span	WAIS-R Digit Span
	Trail Making Test	TMT

[a] The MMSE was used for screening, not as an outcome variable.

assessment consisted of three sessions. The first session began approximately 2 to 3 hours after the subject's arising from sleep, after the subject's return from breakfast, and 5 to 10 minutes after completion of the first MWT. This pattern of neuropsychologic testing and MWT continued until the subject completed the final (fourth) MWT session.

During neuropsychologic testing, subjects were seated comfortably in a well-lit, climate-controlled, sound-attenuated room. A digital, electronic countdown timer was used for tests requiring delay periods, and a similar count-up timer was used for timing tasks.

The testing battery included outcome measures and consisted of eight basic groupings: CVLT, modified WCST, PASAT, Bedside Assessment of Executive Cognitive Impairment (EXIT), Tower of Toronto (TOT), Stroop-color test (Stroop), WAIS-R Digit Span, and TMT.

The Mini Mental State Examination (MMSE), a brief screening instrument for dementia [32], tests orientation, registration, attention, calculation, recall, and language.

The CVLT examines interaction between verbal memory and conceptual ability and evaluates the use and effectiveness of learning strategies [33]. Two shopping lists (16 items each) are presented. Every item belongs to one of four categories. The first list is called the "Monday list." It contains four names of fruits, spices, and herbs, tools, and items of clothing. The subject's task is to recall as many items as possible five times immediately after presentation, two times after a short delay, and two times 20 minutes later. There also is a "Tuesday list," which is presented only once. Delayed recall trials are both unprompted "free recall" and prompted "cued recall." (An example of prompted recall is "Tell me all of the shopping items from the Monday List that are clothing.") The tester notes whether items are recalled by rote or if semantic clusters are used. Incorrect items and repeated correct items are scored as intrusions and perseverations, respectively.

The modified WCST (computerized) measures flexibility in rule formation, often called "abstract behavior" and "shift of set" [34,35]. The test uses 48 cards containing one to four symbols (stars, triangles, crosses, and circles). These symbols appear in red, green, yellow, or blue. Four cards are shown at the top of a computer screen. As each new card appears, the subject must place it under one of the four cards, according to a self-deduced rule. The computer does not explain the rule but rather indicates whether each card placement is correct or incorrect. For example if the rule is color, a correctly placed green card would be under green squares, regardless of the card's symbol or number. The rule changes after six correctly placed cards, and subjects are informed that the rule has changed. This procedure continues until 48 cards are shown or six rule changes are mastered.

The PASAT measures arithmetic computational ability at different speeds [36]. It requires attention and concentration. A prerecorded tape presents 50 one-digit numbers in random order. Subjects must add each sequential pair of numbers. For example, if the first five numbers were 5, 4, 9, 2, and 3, the first four correct responses would be 9, 13, 11, and 5. Four 50-number sequences are presented by audiotape at four rates of speed (2.4, 2.0, 1.6, and 1.2 seconds between digits). This difficult task requires sustained attention with simultaneous inhibition of the subject's own response.

The EXIT measures several factors related to executive functions [37]. Originally designed for clinical bedside use, this test focuses on functional status, problem behaviors engendered, and executive dyscontrol. Separate scores are derived for frontal release, motor or cognitive perseveration, verbal intrusions, disinhibition, loss of spontaneity, imitation behavior, environmental dependency, and use behavior. Each of the 25 items is scored on a three-point basis: 0 indicates intact performance; 1 indicates a specific partial error or equivocal response; 2 indicates a specific incorrect response or failure to perform the task. High interrater reliability ($r = .90$) and correlation with MMSE are reported.

The TOT assesses planning ability and problem solving [38]. Subjects must move three wooden disks of differing size from the initial position (in descending size on the leftmost stick) to a predetermined position on another (in the same order on the rightmost stick). Only one disk may be moved at a time, and a larger disk must not be put on top of a smaller disc. At all times disks must remain on one of the three sticks. The goal is to make as few moves as possible. An analogous but more complex test uses four disks with the same rules and goals.

The Stroop indexes linguistic interference with color naming. It is thought to measure ease and rapidity of shifting from one perceptual set to another [39]. This three-part test requires subjects to read color names (blue, green, and red) and name the colors seen (XXXX's printed in blue, green, or red). On the third trial the colors that must be named are used to print the names of different colors. For example, the word "red" is printed in green, and the correct response is to say "green." Each trial is 45 seconds in duration. This test is sensitive to left frontal lobe dysfunction [40].

The WAIS-R Digit Span is a WAIS subtest [41]. It assesses auditory attention and concentration for numbers and short-term memory [42]. Subjects are asked to repeat numbers in the order of presentation (Digit Span Forward) or in reverse order (Digit Span Backward). Each successive trial increases the number of digits presented until the subject's limit (span) is reached or the subject has completed all rows of numbers (a maximum of nine one-digit numbers in the Digit Span Forward and a maximum of eight in the Digit Span Backward) successfully.

The TMT tests complex visual scanning, letter and number recognition, cognitive flexibility, and perceptual-motor speed. Motor speed and agility contribute to the test outcome [32,43]. The subject must draw lines to connect consecutively numbered circles on one worksheet (part A) and then connect in alternating order the same number of consecutively numbered and lettered circles on another worksheet (part B). Subjects are instructed to connect the circles "as fast as you can." Mistakes are pointed out until the test is completed without mistakes. Scoring is based on time. This test is a sensitive indicator of the presence of nonspecific brain dysfunction [44].

Results

All data were analyzed using SAS/SAT statistical software for Personal Computers, Version 6.04 (SAS Institute, Inc., Cary, North Carolina, 1985). Group comparability testing was performed using student *t*-tests. Neuropsychologic test data were analyzed using General Linear Models Analysis of Variance (GLM) procedures. The basic experimental design was a randomized, parallel group, controlled, repeated measures (before and after treatment) trial.

Group comparability testing

To determine group comparability, important sleep parameters were compared between groups at baseline. Table 3 shows group means and SD for treated and untreated subjects. No group differences were found. The authors further classified CPAP-treated patients on the basis of use. Patients who used the machine for a mean of more than 5 hours per night (based on reading the hour meter during the follow-up visit) were classified as treated compliant (TC). The remainder was classified as treated noncompliant (TNC). Mean apnea index (AI) and AHI were significantly lower ($P < .05$) in the TNC group than in the TC group (see Table 3).

To validate treatment efficacy, AI, AHI, and SaO$_2$ nadir were compared at follow-up between treated and untreated patients. At follow-up, mean AI, AHI, and SaO$_2$ nadirs were 2.36, 5.05, and 88.81%, respectively for the treated group. By contrast, mean AI, AHI, and SaO$_2$ nadirs were 25.82, 39.81, and 77.33% for the untreated group. The treated and untreated groups differed significantly in AI and AHI but not in SaO$_2$ nadir at follow-up. TC and TNC groups (which differed at baseline in AI and AHI) did not differ at follow-up. The untreated group differed significantly from both TC and TNC in these parameters. The SaO$_2$ nadir did not differ between the treated, TC, and TNC groups at follow-up.

Neuropsychologic tests

Sleep studies were tabulated and scored blindly. The overall experimental design can be represented as follows: main effects for group (treated versus untreated); session (baseline versus follow-up); number of subjects to be tested. The interaction effect for group × session provided a test for the differential effect of CPAP therapy on an outcome measure. Additional GLM analyses were conducted with a trifurcated group factor (TC, TCN, and untreated).

California Verbal Learning Test From the CVLT one obtains a great number of scores. These can be grouped as

1. The number of correctly recalled words (from Monday and Tuesday lists)
2. The number of perseverations (repeated words during recall on trials)

Table 3: Sleep parameters at baseline in patients who had obstructive sleep apnea

Variable	U (N = 12) Mean	SD	T (N = 17) Mean	SD	TC (N = 9) Mean	SD	TNC (N = 8) Mean	SD	T vs. U P-value	TC vs. U P-value	TNC vs. U P-value	TNC vs. TC P-value
Apnea index	21.6	19.8	23.5	26.2	36.3	30.4	9.0	7.3	ns	ns	ns	.03
AHI	39.7	25.6	45.5	32.1	60.1	34.3	29.0	20.7	ns	ns	ns	.04
Longest apnea (sec)	52.4	23.5	53.0	23.8	55.7	24.6	49.9	24.2	ns	ns	ns	ns
SaO₂ nadir (%)	78.0	14.7	69.5	20.4	64.3	17.5	75.3	23.0	ns	ns	ns	ns
PLM index	27.0	36.5	23.5	42.0	29.5	53.3	16.7	26.2	ns	ns	ns	ns
PLM arousal index	9.7	11.3	8.0	14.6	7.5	16.0	8.7	13.9	ns	ns	ns	ns

Abbreviations: AHI, apnea-hypopnea index; ns, not significant; PLM, periodic leg movement; SaO₂, arterial oxygen saturation; T, treated; TC, treated compliant; TNC, treated noncompliant; U, untreated.

3. The number of intrusions (incorrect words other than perseverations on trials)
4. Words recalled using learning strategies

Learning strategies include serial clustering (recall in order, matching initial presentation) and semantic clustering (recall using linguistically meaningful categories). No CPAP-related improvements were found on any individual trial of CVLT for the number of correctly recalled words, intrusions, perseverations, or recalled words using learning strategies (serial or semantic clustering) on the Monday list (see Table 4). Two CPAP-related declines were noted: perseverations on trial 1 and serial clustering on the delayed free recall of words on the Monday list. No CPAP-related differences were found between treated and untreated patients for the mean, maximum, or minimum number of correctly recalled words, perseverations, intrusions, or number of words recalled using learning strategies (semantic or serial clustering) across all trials on the Monday list. Similarly, CPAP-related differences were not found for proactive or retroactive interference between Monday and Tuesday list recall. Analyses also were conducted taking CPAP usage into account. No additional CPAP-related differences were found on any Monday list parameter when use was used to stratify groups. Significant group × session differences were found for the Tuesday list, however. Further analysis taking CPAP usage into account revealed that patients in the TC group did not have perseverations at either baseline or follow-up; therefore, the patients in the TNC group produced the locus of change. Fig. 1 shows results from the trial with the Tuesday list. A significant CPAP-related decline in perseverations was found. Other parameters (number of correctly recalled words and intrusions and number recalled using semantic or serial clustering [not shown]) did not differ significantly.

Wisconsin Card Sorting Test Robust practice effects were observed for the number of correct and number of perseverations on WCST; however, no CPAP-related improvement in any parameter was found (see Table 4). Furthermore, CPAP-use analysis yielded no significant findings.

Paced Auditory Serial Addition Task Table 4 shows the combined mean scores (sum of trials 1–4/4) for treated and untreated groups at baseline and follow-up. The analysis reveals an overall significant effect for session. After adjusting for practice, however, no significant differences between groups were found. Although there were no CPAP-related differences for means across trials, treatment-related differences were found in several individual trials (differing in presentation speed).

Table 4: Neuropsychologic test for treated and untreated groups

Test	Variable	S	T (N = 17) Mean	SD	U (N = 12) Mean	SD	Group Difference P-value	Group × Session P-value	Session Effect P-value
CVLT	Mean number of correct responses across trials	1	8.5	1.9	9.2	2.2	ns	ns	.0001
		2	10.3	1.7	10.7	2.8	ns		
	Mean number of perseverations across trials	1	0.8	0.7	0.7	0.7	ns	ns	.0121
		2	0.8	0.7	1.2	1.1	ns		
	Mean number of intrusions across trials	1	0.5	0.5	0.3	0.3	ns	ns	ns
		2	0.5	0.5	0.4	0.4	ns		
WCST	Number correct	1	29.0	9.2	25.4	11.4	ns	ns	.008
		2	34.1	5.4	29.7	11.4	ns		
	Number of errors	1	12.2	6.5	9.1	5.5	ns	ns	.054
		2	9.1	5.5	11.0	7.5	ns		
	Number of perseverations	1	5.1	6.8	9.3	12.8	ns	ns	.090
		2	3.0	4.6	6.5	11.3	ns		
PASAT	Mean number of correct responses	1	115.5	29.3	122.7	27.7	ns	ns	.0001
		2	130.4	31.0	133.6	27.1	ns		
	Mean number of errors	1	16.0	11.1	20.8	13.3	ns	ns	.0002
		2	11.2	9.5	12.8	8.6	ns		
	Mean number of omissions	1	63.6	30.8	52.4	24.8	ns	ns	.0018
		2	53.9	29.5	49.1	25.8	ns		
EXIT	Mean score	1	6.2	3.3	5.5	3.2	ns	ns	.056
		2	4.9	2.8	4.5	1.6	ns		
STROOP	Word reading: number of words	1	75.8	18.7	84.7	16.1	ns	ns	ns
		2	77.8	17.5	83.9	16.0	ns		
	Color Naming: number of words	1	56.6	13.1	69.4	12.7	0.014	ns	ns
		2	58.8	12.1	68.5	11.9	0.042		
	Colored word naming: number of words	1	28.5	7.1	32.6	9.4	ns	ns	.001
		2	31.3	9.3	36.5	7.0	ns		
WAIS-R	Forward digit span	1	7.8	2.4	7.1	1.8	ns	0.007	.001
		2	8.0	2.5	8.7	2.2	ns		
	Backward digit span	1	6.2	2.3	5.9	2.6	ns	ns	ns
		2	6.4	2.0	6.5	2.1	ns		
TMT	TRAILS-A	1	38.4	12.8	32.1	9.7	ns	0.051	.034
		2	31.2	10.9	31.8	6.5	ns		
	TRAILS-B	1	87.4	29.4	91.8	50.6	ns	ns	.025
		2	75.5	38.3	72.3	21.7	ns		

Abbreviations: CVLT, California Verbal Learning Test; EXIT, Bedside Assessment of Executive Cognitive Impairment-Executive Interview; ns, not significant; PASAT, Paced Auditory Serial Addition Task; S, session; STROOP, Stroop Color-Word Test; T, treated; TMT, Trail-making Test; U, untreated; WAIS-R, Wechsler Adult Intelligence Scale–revised; WCST, Modified Wisconsin Card-sorting Test; 1, baseline; 2, follow-up.

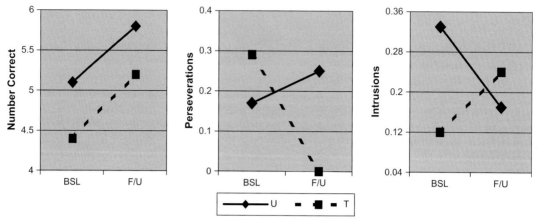

Fig. 1. California Verbal Learning Test Tuesday list: number of correct responses, perseverations, and intrusions for treated and untreated groups at baseline (BSL) and follow-up (F/U). Significant CPAP-related group differences were found for number of perseverations (P = .05).

Group × session interaction was found for the number of errors (P < .04) and omissions (P < .02) on trials with 2-second intervals. A slightly different pattern of results emerges when CPAP usage is taken into account. Fig. 2 shows an overall significant effect for session on all test parameters (number of correct responses, number of errors, and number of omissions). After adjustment for practice, a significant group × session interaction (P = .040) was found for the mean number of omissions, with a dramatic decrease in the TC group but only a slight decline in the TNC and untreated groups (7, 1.5, and 3 for the TC, TNC, and untreated groups, respectively), even though there were no significant differences between groups at baseline. In summary, the PASAT lends partial support to the hypothesis that CPAP improves cognitive ability. The number of correct additions and

the number of errors seem to be insensitive to treatment. By contrast, the number of omissions declined differentially across groups, reaching significance on trials 2 and 4, and in the totals when treatment use was considered. Therefore, the number of omissions may provide some limited outcome index related to treatment efficacy in attention and concentration.

Bedside Assessment of Executive Cognitive Impairment   No significant CPAP-related changes were found on the EXIT, regardless of whether the treated group is compared with the untreated group or whether CPAP usage is considered in the analysis (see Table 4). Scores on this test revealed a near ceiling effect in responding.

Tower of Toronto   Tower of Toronto has trials using three disks (TOT3) and four disks (TOT4).

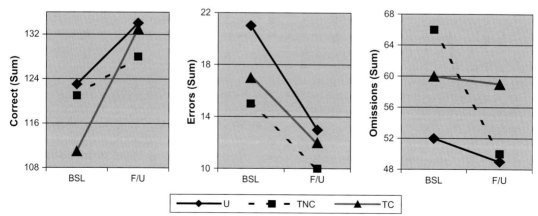

Fig. 2. Paced Auditory Serial Addition Task (across trials): number of correct responses, errors, and omissions for untreated (U), treated compliant (TC), and treated noncompliant (TNC) groups at baseline (BSL) and follow-up (F/U). Significant CPAP-related group differences were found for omissions (P = .001) and nearly significant differences were found for correct responses (P = .051).

Table 5: Tower of Toronto 3 and 4: outcomes for treated and untreated groups

Test	Variable	S	T (N = 17) Mean	SD	U (N = 12) Mean	SD	Group Difference P-value	Group × Session P-value	Session Effect P-value
TOT3	Trial 1: number of moves	1	10.8	5.7	10.3	3.7	ns	ns	ns
		2	7.8	1.7	8.7	4.7	ns		.006
	Trial 1: number of violations	1	0.7	1.1	0.5	0.8	ns	ns	ns
		2	0.0	0.0	0.2	0.4	ns		
	Trial 2: number of moves	1	8.1	2.0	8.4	2.0	ns	ns	ns
		2	8.2	2.8	8.3	3.3	ns		.087
	Trial 2: number of violations	1	0.0	0.0	0.2	0.4	ns	.087	.087
		2	0.0	0.0	0.0	0.0	na		
	Trial 3: number of moves	1	8.3	2.7	8.9	3.6	ns	ns	ns
		2	8.1	3.4	7.6	2.0	ns		
	Trial 3: number of violations	1	8.3	2.7	8.9	3.6	ns	ns	ns
		2	8.1	3.4	7.6	2.0	na		
TOT4	Trial 1: number of moves	1	42.8	24.8	26.8	13.2	.035	ns	.086
		2	26.7	16.6	25.5	9.7	ns		
	Trial 1: number of violations	1	0.8	1.0	1.3	2.8	ns	.019	ns
		2	0.1	0.3	0.3	0.8	ns		
	Trial 2: number of moves	1	25.9	9.9	30.2	16.7	ns	ns	ns
		2	22.3	7.6	28.0	12.8	ns		
	Trial 2: number of violations	1	0.2	0.6	0.6	1.4	ns	ns	ns
		2	0.0	0.0	0.3	1.2	ns		
	Trial 3: number of moves	1	27.8	13.6	27.4	14.4	ns	ns	ns
		2	21.9	9.3	28.8	13.5	ns		
	Trial 3: number of violations	1	0.2	0.5	0.1	0.3	ns	ns	ns
		2	0.0	0.0	0.1	0.3	ns		
	Trial 4: number of moves	1	26.2	11.9	25.1	14.7	ns	ns	ns
		2	22.8	9.2	24.6	9.2	ns		
	Trial 4: number of violations	1	0.1	0.5	0.4	0.7	ns	ns	.019
		2	0.0	0.0	0.0	0.0	na		

Abbreviations: ns, not significant; S, session; T, treated; TOT, Tower of Toronto; U, untreated.

Results are shown in Table 5. After adjustment for practice effects, no significant differences between groups were found. There was, however, a trend in the number of violations in trial 2 ($P = .087$). The mean number of errors decreased more in the untreated group than in the treated group. The treated group could not show any decrease in mean numbers of violations, having had zero at baseline. A ceiling effect is probably operative here, because the best score (ie, fewest moves) is 7; the mean maximum of moves was 11.29 (SD, 5.53) in the treated group and 11.00 (SD, 5.63) in the untreated group. For the four-disk TOT, the untreated group had a greater decrease in violations than the treated group (0.92 violations versus 0.70 violations). This result goes against the investigators' predictions and remains difficult to explain. Groups did not differ significantly at baseline.

These data show that after adjusting for practice effects, no significant CPAP-related improvement was found in planning abilities as assessed by the TOT3 or TOT4. Analyses were also conducted taking CPAP usage into account and did not reveal any additional CPAP-related differences.

Stroop-color test   No significant CPAP-related changes were found on Stroop, regardless of whether the treated group is compared with the untreated group or whether CPAP usage was considered in the analysis (see Table 4). Significant practice effects were seen, however.

Wechsler Adult Intelligence Scale–Revised Digit Span   Practice effect was found on Digit Span Forward ($P = .001$). Surprisingly, the untreated group improved more than the treated group ($P = .007$) when baseline was compared with follow-up (see Table 4). This unexpected finding is contrary to the investigators' expectations. On analyses taking CPAP usage into account, the same opposite effect

was found, with the TC group worsening and the untreated and TNC groups improving.

Trail-making Test   A near significant CPAP-related improvement was found for the TMT-A ($P = .051$). The mean number of seconds decreased less in the untreated group than in the treated group (7.11 seconds versus 0.33 seconds). There was a trend for untreated group to be faster (6.27 seconds) than the treated group at baseline (Fig. 3). When CPAP use was taken into account, no significant differences between groups or trends were found.

Discussion

The results of this study indicate that few CPAP-related improvements occur on a restricted number of neuropsychologic tests. The investigators found significantly decreased ($P < .05$) perseverations on the CVLT Tuesday list, decreased omissions on the PASAT (sum, $P = .001$; trial 2, $P = .016$; trial 4, $P = .040$), fewer violations on the four-disk TOT (trial 2, $P = .087$), and near-significant ($P = .051$) improvement on the TMT-A. No other significant improvements beyond practice were found for any other measures on the CVLT, modified WCST, PASAT, EXIT, TOT, Stroop, WAIS–Revised Digit Span, and TMT. By contrast, practice effects were robust and pervasive. With few exceptions, subjects improved at session 2 regardless of their treatment or CPAP use status. This finding underscores the absolute necessity for CPAP outcome trials to include a randomized, parallel control group as part of the design. The results largely agree with a controlled study performed by Bardwell and colleagues [45] who administered the WAIS-Revised Digit Symbol and Digit Span, TMT A/B, Digit Vigilance, Stroop, Digit Ordering, and Word Fluency tests before

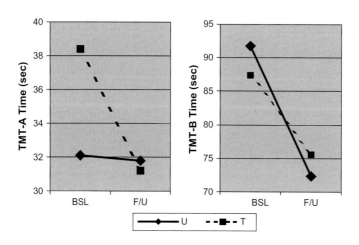

Fig. 3. Trail-making Test (Trails-A and Trails-B) for treated and untreated groups at baseline (BSL) and follow-up (F/U). A CPAP-related nearly significant difference ($P = .051$) was found for Trails-A.

and after CPAP therapy [45]. They found improvement on only 1 of 22 measures generated by their neuropsychologic test battery. Similarly, another study in which baseline differences were noted did not find CPAP-related improvements when compared with a sham-CPAP control [46].

The authors' test selection was determined partially by a desire to explore the relationship between sleepiness and executive function. Studies of total sleep deprivation indicate deterioration in higher cognitive abilities after 36 hours. Word fluency, word inhibition, and nonverbal tasks measuring flexibility and planning are sensitive to sleep loss; critical reasoning is not impaired, however [47]. Similarly, Binks and colleagues [48] report no changes in higher cortical functions after 34 to 36 hours of sleep deprivation. Their test battery included the PASAT, Stroop (Victoria version), WCST, WAIS-R IQ, Category Test (Booklet Form), Word Fluency Test, and the Shipley Scale. Similarly, in a study of patients who had sleep apnea, diminished baseline function on visuospatial learning and motor performance returned to normal after CPAP therapy, but sustained attention, executive function, and constructional abilities did not improve even after 4 months [49].

One explanation for a lack of CPAP-related neuropsychologic improvements is that OSA is marked by partial, not total, sleep deprivation. Typically, in OSA sleep disturbance is caused mainly to fragmentation. The intervening sleep, although not consolidated, may allow cognitive abilities to remain intact. Patients may become sleepy, fatigued, irritable, and distractible; however, the sleep deprivation is partial and evolves gradually. Thus, adaptations may occur. That is, patients may develop coping strategies that allow for "best effort" performance within a time-limited domain. Furthermore, an individual may accept limitations and cease attempting certain activities. Under such circumstances one would not expect much deficit and consequently no improvement on neuropsychologic tests. In fact, Verstraeten and colleagues [50] argue that the slowing of information processing and disruption in short-term memory are key. They point out that their results indicated no deficits/improvements in disinhibition, distractibility, preservation, attention switching, or working memory. By contrast, Aloia and cowokers [51] find improved executive function and attention in addition to motor speed and recall when CPAP therapeutic adherence is taken into consideration.

Another explanation relates to linguistic ambiguity in self-reporting. For example, patients frequently complain about having "difficulty remembering things." One possibility is that different aspects of memory are affected differentially by sleep apnea or are restored differentially by treatment [52]. Another possibility is that clinicians focus on the words "remembering things," interpreting this statement to mean that memory impairment has developed. The key word in the patient's message, however, may be "difficulty." If the patient's message is difficulty, not memory, then test performance will not indicate impairment unless the task requirements exceed the patient's overall ability. Cognitive and psychomotor slowing often occurs with sleep loss and in sleep-deprived individuals [53]. In such instances, when performance is overtaxed, test outcome may suffer as a result of slowing (eg, the decreased number of omissions in the treated group on the PASAT). Therefore, if difficulty is the issue, increased effort may compensate for slowing, thereby enabling normal or near-normal levels of performance. Most controlled studies (including the present study) find little or no improvements in test of performance. Experimental paradigms in this field of inquiry, however, do not consider or measure effort during performance. As such, potential CPAP-related improvements (ie, a decrease in the effort required) may go unnoticed.

By contrast, the paucity of findings may reflect simply a differential time course for sleepiness, mood, and cognitive improvement related to CPAP therapy. Self-reported sleepiness improves within the first week of treatment [18]. Mood improves within 3 weeks [16,22]. Randomized CPAP trials vary with respect to the interval between treatment initiation and follow-up testing. Bailey [20] reports no improvement in neuropsychologic test scores (except visual memory) at 3 days. Similarly, Bardwell and colleagues [23] found no change at 10 days, and Brown [16,18] found little change at 3 weeks (namely, finger tapping and short-term memory). By contrast, at a mean of 16.6 days to follow-up, Froeling and coworkers [24] report improved Rey Auditory Verbal Learning, Grooved Pegboard, PASAT, and Stroop scores. The authors did not find such pervasive improvement after approximately 2 weeks of CPAP therapy but confirmed PASAT improvement. The longest reported treatment period in any study was 3 months. At 3 months, with good CPAP use (5.9 hours per night), Engleman and colleagues [21] failed to show treatment-related improvement in neuropsychologic function on any of the seven tests in their battery. Nonetheless, this finding does not rule out the possibility that even more time is required to see significant cognitive improvement.

Most standardized neuropsychologic tests seem to be insensitive to CPAP treatment outcome. This conclusion was also reached by Lojander and colleagues [54] based on their neuropsychologic testing of patients who had sleep-disordered breathing before, after 3 months, and after 1 year of treatment with CPAP, surgery, or conservative (control) therapy. Statistically the authors' failure to find treatment-related differences may have resulted from the study being underpowered. If such were the case, however, they would expect to see consistent trends. Many of these tests were designed to detect, localize, or diagnose brain lesions or damage. One might argue that the lack of findings provide test validation that the scores are largely unaltered by functional, reversible conditions. It remains to be determined if there actually is CPAP-related improvement in cognitive or executive ability. The challenge for the future, assuming that there is such improvement, will be to develop more sensitive techniques for measuring such changes. The paradigms currently in use seem inadequate to produce reliable and consistent findings. Motor speed, auditory serial addition (at a fairly rapid pace), trail making, and memory seem likely candidates for further exploration. Incorporating indices for the amount of effort applied by subjects during test performance may prove useful for understanding CPAP-related changes. As clinicians, the authors' believe that reported cognitive improvement after treatment has some basis in fact. Using standard testing instruments, however, they find little measurable change. Further large-scale studies, like the ongoing multicenter APPLES project, are required to resolve this paradox.

References

[1] Guilleminault C, Partinen MD, Quera-Salva MA, et al. Determinants of daytime sleepiness in obstructive sleep apnea. Chest 1988;9:32–7.

[2] Sackner MA, Landa J, Forrest T, et al. Periodic sleep apnea: chronic sleep deprivation related to intermittent upper airway obstruction and central nervous system disturbance. Chest 1975; 67:164–71.

[3] Millman RP, Fogel BS, McNamara ME, et al. Depression as a manifestation of obstructive sleep apnea: reversal with nasal continuous positive airway pressure. J Clin Psychiatry 1989;50:348–51.

[4] Flemons WW, Tsai W. Quality of life consequences of sleep-disordered breathing. J Allergy Clin Immunol 1997;99:750–6.

[5] Cheshire K, Engleman H, Deary I, et al. Factors impairing daytime performance in patients with sleep apnea/hypopnea syndrome. Arch Intern Med 1992;152:538–41.

[6] Redline S, Strauss ME, Adams N, et al. Neuropsychological function in mild sleep disordered breathing. Sleep 1997;20:160–7.

[7] Orth M, Duchna HW, Leidag M, et al. Driving simulator and neuropsychological testing in OSAS before and under CPAP therapy. Eur Respir J 2005;26(5):898–903.

[8] Adams N, Strauss M, Schluchter M, et al. Relation of measures of sleep-disordered breathing to neuropsychological functioning. Am J Respir Crit Care Med 2001;163(7):1626–31.

[9] Greenberg GD, Watson RK, Deptula D. Neuropsychological dysfunction in sleep apnea. Sleep 1987;10:254–62.

[10] Findley L, Barth JT, Powers DC, et al. Cognitive impairment in patients with obstructive sleep apnea and associated hypoxemia. Chest 1986;90:686–90.

[11] Dealberto MJ, Pajot N, Curbon D, et al. Breathing disorders during sleep and cognitive performance in an older community sample: the EVA Study. J Am Geriatr Soc 1996;44:1287–94.

[12] Guilleminault C. Clinical features and evaluation of obstructive sleep apnea. In: Kryger MH, Roth T, Dement WC, editors. Principles and practice of sleep medicine. 2nd edition. Philadelphia: Saunders; 1994. p. 667–78.

[13] Naëgelé B, Thouvard V, Péping JL, et al. Deficits of cognitive executive functions in patients with sleep apnea syndrome. Sleep 1995;18:43–52.

[14] Naëgelé B, Pepin J-L, Levy P, Bonnet C, et al. Cognitive executive dysfunction in patients with obstructive sleep apnea syndrome (OSAS) after CPAP treatment. Sleep 1998;21:392–7.

[15] Ingram F, Henke KG, Levin HS, et al. Sleep apnea and vigilance performance in a community-dwelling older sample. Sleep 1994;17:248–52.

[16] Lee MM, Strauss ME, Adams N, et al. Executive functions in persons with sleep apnea. Sleep Breath 1999;3:13–6.

[17] Bédard MA, Montplaisir J, Malo J, et al. Persistent neuropsychological deficits and vigilance impairment in sleep apnea syndrome after treatment with continuous positive airways pressure (CPAP). J Clin Exp Neuropsychol 1993;15: 330–41.

[18] Brown WD, Jamieson AO, Becker PM, et al. Cognitive, emotional and behavioral correlates of obstructive sleep apnea and the effects of continuous positive airway pressure (CPAP) treatment: the importance of a control group. Sleep Research 1991;20:213.

[19] Mendelson BW, Maczaj M, Putnam K, et al. cognitive measures in obstructive sleep apnea patients before and after treatment. Sleep Research 1993; 22:235.

[20] Bailey GL. Neuropsychological functioning, sleep and vigilance in men with obstructive sleep apnea syndrome treated with continuous positive airway pressure [dissertation]. Tallahassee (FL): Florida State University; 1993.

[21] Engleman HM, Cheshire KE, Deary IJ, et al. Daytime sleepiness, cognitive performance and mood after continuous positive airway pressure for the sleep apnoea/hypopnoea syndrome. Thorax 1993;48:911–4.

[22] Engleman HM, Kingshott RN, Wraith PK, et al. Randomized placebo-controlled crossover trial

of continuous positive airway pressure for mild sleep apnea/hypopnea syndrome. Am J Resp Crit Care Med 1999;159:461–7.

[23] Bardwell WA, Ancoli-Israel S, Dimsdale JE. Neuropsychological effects of continuous positive airway pressure treatment in patients with obstructive sleep apnea: a placebo-controlled study. Sleep 1999;22:S29.

[24] Froehling B, Seidenberg M, Georgemiller R, et al. Neuropsychological and affective dysfunction in sleep apnea syndrome: response to nasal continuous positive airway pressure treatment. Sleep Research 1991;20:244.

[25] Boland LL, Shahar E, Iber C, et al. Measures of cognitive function in persons with varying degrees of sleep-disordered breathing: the Sleep Heart Health Study. J Sleep Res 2002;11(3):265–72.

[26] Reynolds CF, Kupfer DJ, McEachran AB, et al. Depressive psychopathology in male sleep apneics. J Clin Psychiatry 1984;45:287–90.

[27] Derman S, Karacan I. Sleep-induced respiratory disorders. Psychiatr Ann 1979;9:411–25.

[28] Douglass AB, Bornstein R, Nino-Murcia G, et al. The sleep disorders questionnaire I: creation and multivariate structure of SDQ. Sleep 1994;17:160–7.

[29] Rechtschaffen A, Kales A. A manual of standardized, techniques and scoring system for sleep stages in human subjects. NIH Publication # 204. Washington, DC: National Institutes of Health; 1968.

[30] Bornstein SK. Respiratory monitoring during sleep: polysomnography. In: Guilleminault C, editor. Sleeping and waking disorders: indications and techniques. Menlo Park (CA): Addison-Wesley; 1982. p. 183–212.

[31] Bonnet M, Carley D, Guilleminault C, et al. Recording and scoring leg movements. Sleep 1993;16:748–59.

[32] Folstein MF, Folstein SE, McHugh PR. Minimental state. J Psychiatr Res 1975;12:189–98.

[33] Delis DL, Kramer JH, Kaplan E, et al. California Verbal Learning Test Adult Version. San Antonio (TX): The Psychological Corporation; 1987.

[34] Nelson HE. A modified card sorting test sensitive to frontal lobe defects. Cortex 1976;12:313–24.

[35] Lezak DM. Neuropsychological assessment. 3rd edition. New York: Oxford University Press; 1995.

[36] Gronwall DMA. Paced Auditory Serial-Addition Task: a measure of recovery from concussion. Percept Mot Skills 1977;44:367–73.

[37] Royall DR, Mahurin RK, Gray KF. Bedside Assessment of Executive Cognitive Impairment. The executive interview. J Clin Exp Neuropsychol 1992;12:1221–6.

[38] Glosser G, Goodglass H. Disorders in executive control functions among aphasic and other brain-damaged patients. J Clin Exp Neuropsychol 1990;12:485–501.

[39] Thurstone LL, Mellinger JJ. The Stroop Test. Raleigh (NC): The Psychometric Laboratory of the University of North Carolina; 1953.

[40] Golden JC. Identification of brain disorder by the Stroop Color-Word Test. J Clin Psychol 1976;32:654–8.

[41] Wechsler D. Wechsler Adult Intelligence Scale–Revised manual. New York: Psychological Corporation; 1981.

[42] Sattler JM. Assessment of children. San Diego (CA): Sattler Publishing; 1988.

[43] Reitan RM. Validity of the Trail Making Test as an indication of organic brain injury. Percept Mot Skills 1958;8:271–6.

[44] Spreen O, Bentson AL. Comparative studies of some psychological tests for cerebral damage. J Nerv Ment Dis 1965;140:323–33.

[45] Bardwell WA, Ancoli-Israel S, Berry CC, et al. Neuropsychological effects of one-week continuous positive airway pressure treatment in patients with obstructive sleep apnea: a placebo-controlled study. Psychosom Med 2001;63(4):579–84.

[46] Henke KG, Grady JJ, Kuna ST. Effect of nasal continuous positive airway pressure on neuropsychological function in sleep apnea-hypopnea syndrome. A randomized, placebo-controlled trial. Am J Respir Crit Care Med 2001;163(4):911–7.

[47] Horne J. Frontal lobe function and sleep loss. Sleep Res, in press.

[48] Binks GP, Waters FW, Hurry M. Short-term total sleep deprivations does not selectively impair higher cortical functioning. Sleep 1999;22:328–34.

[49] Ferini-Strambi L, Baietto C, Di Gioia MR, et al. Cognitive dysfunction in patients with obstructive sleep apnea (OSA): partial reversibility after continuous positive airway pressure (CPAP). Brain Res Bull 2003;61(1):87–92.

[50] Verstraeten E, Cluydts R, Pevernagie D, et al. Executive function in sleep apnea: controlling for attentional capacity in assessing executive attention. Sleep 2004;27:685–93.

[51] Aloia MS, Ilniczky N, Di Dio P, et al. Neuropsychological changes and treatment compliance in older adults with sleep apnea. J Psychosom Res 2003;54(1):71–6.

[52] Naegele B, Launois SH, Mazza S, et al. Which memory processes are affected in patients with obstructive sleep apnea? An evaluation of 3 types of memory. Sleep 2006;29(4):533–44.

[53] Dinges D. Proving the limits of functional capability: the effects of sleep loss on short-duration tasks. In: Broughton RJ, Ogilvie RD, editors. Sleep, arousal, and performance. Boston: Birkhauser; 1992. p. 177–88.

[54] Lojander J, Kajaste S, Maasilta P, et al. Cognitive function and treatment of obstructive sleep apnea syndrome. J Sleep Res 1999;8(1):71–6.

ELSEVIER
SAUNDERS

SLEEP
MEDICINE
CLINICS

Sleep Med Clin 1 (2006) 513–517

Sleep-Related Breathing Disorders and Mood Disorders

Ali M. Hashmi, MD[a,b], Nilgun Giray, MD[a,b], Max Hirshkowitz, PhD, D ABSM[a,b],*

- Overview
- Methods
  - Subjects
  - Apparatus and procedures
- Results
- Discussion
- References

It is well recognized that sleepiness results from sleep-disordered breathing (SDB). Many patients who have SDB also show depressive features [1–4]. Other sequelae of SDB include paranoia and personality changes [5], impaired cognitive abilities [6], cognitive complaints [7], and impaired performance on vigilance tests [1,8]. Coleman and colleagues [9] reported one third of patients presenting with insomnia at sleep disorders centers had psychiatric-related sleep problems. Moreover, half of these patients had major depressive disorders. Flemons and Tsai [10] found that patients who have SDB have impaired quality of life, impaired work efficiency, and more automobile accidents. Effectively treating SDB can improve mood, both subjectively [11] and objectively [2,12]. Additionally, sleep studies may be useful for diagnosing occult affective-depressive disorders [13]. Sleepiness affects general health, quality of life, and the self-perception of energy level measured with the medical outcomes survey [14].

Millman and colleagues [2] carefully examined the relationship between SDB and symptoms of depression. Using the Zung Self-Rating Depression Scale, they found a relationship between severity of depression and SDB indices. The apnea plus hypopnea index (AHI) for patients who had Zung scores indicating depression (≥ 50) were compared with indices from patients who had lower depression scores. Mean AHI was significantly higher for patients who had depression (68.0 and 47.9 for depressed and nondepressed patients, respectively). Improved mood was found among patients who had depression treated with nasal continuous positive airway pressure but not for those who had subclinical baseline scores for depression. These authors conclude that SDB can produce symptoms of depression related to apnea severity, and treating the breathing disorder often can alleviate the depression.

Attempts also have been made to determine whether the incidence of depression varies in patients who have and do not have sleep apnea [15]. In a study of 42 patients diagnosed as having SDB (AHI > 15 events/hour), 26% had depression indicated by Beck Depression Inventory (BDI) scores of 13 or more. An additional 22 patients were found to have fewer than 15 breathing events

[a] Baylor College of Medicine, 1 Baylor Plaza, Houston, TX 77030, USA
[b] Sleep Disorders & Research Center, Michael E. DeBakey Veterans Affairs Medical Center (111i), 2002 Holcombe Blvd., Houston, TX 77030, USA
* Corresponding author. Sleep Center (111i), 2002 Holcombe Blvd,. Bldg. 100, Rm 6C344, Houston, TX 77030.
E-mail address: maxh@bcm.tmc.edu (M. Hirshkowitz).

doi:10.1016/j.jsmc.2006.11.001

per hour; their depression scores were significantly higher than the group of patients who had sleep apnea syndrome. Polysomnographic information concerning sleep continuity, integrity, and architecture were not reported. These authors conclude that clinical suspicion for depression should be high in patients presenting with symptoms suggesting sleep apnea in whom sleep studies do not reveal significant SDB.

This study examines the relationship between measures of self-reported sleepiness, depressive symptoms, and sleep architecture in a group of patients diagnosed as having obstructive sleep apnea. SDB and depression are comorbid in a significant percentage of patients, but it is unclear how often depression is pre-existent (primary) or an exhaustion-related sequela to the SDB (secondary). On the basis of previous research, the authors hypothesized that a relationship exists between depression as measured by the BDI and the severity of SDB. They also question whether excessive sleepiness and depressive symptoms correlate. Finally, they seek to determine the relationship, if any, between depressive symptoms and measures of sleep continuity, integrity, and architecture.

Methods

Subjects

Ninety-eight subjects were included in the present study. All subjects were male veterans referred for evaluation of sleep-related breathing impairment. Subjects were evaluated with polysomnography and diagnosed as having obstructive sleep apnea according to International Classification of Sleep Disorders criteria [13]. Means and SD for age, body mass index, apnea index (AI), AHI, and saturated arterial oxygen (SaO_2) nadir are shown in Table 1.

Apparatus and procedures

As part of their clinical evaluation, subjects are administered a questionnaire battery that includes the Epworth Sleepiness Scale (ESS) and BDI. The BDI [16] is widely used to assess mood associated

with depression. It is designed for use with both psychiatric patients and normal individuals. Twenty-one symptoms are evaluated; respondents rate the intensity of each symptom on a four-point scale. For example, individuals are asked to rate their sense of failure, guilt feelings, irritability, sleep disturbances, and loss of appetite. Total scores indicate general depression level. The inventory is self-administered and takes 5 to 10 minutes to complete. Reliability and validity studies demonstrate the BDI's effectiveness for indexing mood disorders. The ESS [17] is a widely used, reliable method for measuring persistent daytime sleepiness in adults. It is a self-administered eight-item questionnaire that addresses the patient's self-reported probability of dozing in eight hypothetical settings. The assessment scale ranges from 0 to 3 (0 = would never doze; 1 = slight chance of dosing; 2 = moderate chance of dosing; and 3 = high chance of dozing). The hypothetical settings are

1. Sitting and reading
2. Watching television
3. Sitting, inactive in a public place (eg, a theater or a meeting)
4. Riding as a passenger in a car for an hour without a break
5. Lying down to rest in the afternoon when circumstances permit
6. Sitting and talking to someone
7. Sitting quietly after a lunch without alcohol
8. Sitting in a car while stopped for a few minutes in traffic

Each subject also had undergone attended, laboratory-based, comprehensive polysomnography with continuous recording of monopolar electroencephalograms from central and occipital derivations (C3 or C4 and O3 or O4), electro-oculograms from left and right eye, submentalis (chin) electromyograms, anterior tibialis electromyograms (both legs), modified precordial ECG, nasal-oral airflow, respiratory effort, and SaO_2. Body position also was noted. The authors attempted to schedule bedtimes and morning awakening times to resemble the patient's usual habit. Patients reported to the laboratory approximately 1 hour before scheduled bedtime to complete presleep questionnaires and have monitoring devices attached by a trained technologist. During the day before the study, patients maintained their usual sleep and exercise habits and were instructed to abstain from alcoholic beverages, naps, and caffeinated beverages and meals after 5 PM. A presleep questionnaire provided information on adherence to these restrictions.

Recording and scoring techniques followed currently published recommendations for human

Table 1: Age, body mass index and sleep-disordered breathing

Variable	Mean	SD
Age (years)	53.2	10.1
Body mass index (kg/m²)	35.4	6.8
Apnea index (events/hr sleep)	20.5	20.5
Apnea-hypopnea index (events/hr sleep)	43.5	29.8
SaO_2 nadir (%)	72.8	14.5

subjects, which include procedures for sleep stages [18], arousals [19], respiration [20], and leg movement [21]. In the morning, the monitoring devices were removed, and patients completed a postsleep questionnaire concerning their impression of sleep quantity, quality, and disturbance.

Results

Of the 98 subjects sampled, 35 (35.7%) had BDI total scores of 15 or more. The group mean for the BDI total was 13.6 (SD, 11.3) with a range from 0 to 46. The distribution of BDI total scores is illustrated in Fig. 1. The figure reveals a principle mode of scores ranging from 5 to 9 and a secondary peak at scores ranging from 30 to 34. Table 2 shows the distribution (in percent) of responses on each item of the BDI and characterizes each item. Ten percent of subjects gave the highest rating to items 6 (feeling of being punished), 10 (crying), 16 (sleep disturbance), 17 (tiredness), and 19 (weight loss). Questions on which 20% or more subjects responded with either the highest or second-highest rating included items 13 (difficulty making decisions), 15 (difficulty working), 21 (loss of sexual interest), and 16, 17, and 19.

No correlation was found between BDI total and AI, AHI, or SaO_2 nadir. Similarly, no individual BDI tem correlated with AI or AHI. A solitary correlation was found between item 16's rating of

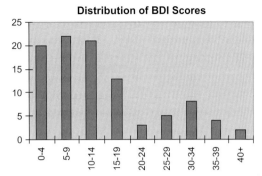

Distribution of BDI Scores

Fig. 1. Percentage distribution of BDI scores. Total scores on the BDI are grouped in intervals of 5 between 0 and 40, showing peaks at 5 to 9 and 30 to 34. BDI scores were in the clinically significant range ($\geq$15) for 37.5% of patients.

sleep disturbance and minimum SaO_2 (r = 0.306; P < .0098). By contrast, the average apnea duration and the duration of the longest apnea episode showed some relationship to BDI scores. Significant negative correlations (P < .05) were found between items 3, 5, 7, and 8, and BDI total and average apnea duration. Marginal negative associations (.05 < P < .10) were found for average apnea duration and items 6 and 19. Longest duration of an apnea episode was significantly related (inversely) with item 8 and marginally with items 3, 15, 19, and BDI total.

Table 2: Percentage distributions for individual Beck Depression Inventory items

Item	Item Characterization	0	1	2	3
01	sadness	60.2	23.5	9.2	7.1
02	discouraged about future	61.2	21.4	8.2	9.2
03	feelings of failure	67.3	15.3	12.2	5.1
04	lack of satisfaction	33.7	49.0	9.2	8.2
05	guilt	74.5	14.3	9.2	2.0
06	feelings of being punished	68.4	13.3	1.0	17.3
07	self disappointment	57.1	31.6	9.2	2.0
08	self blame	50.0	35.7	9.2	5.1
09	suicidal thoughts	68.4	27.6	3.1	1.0
10	crying	59.2	26.5	0.0	14.3
11	irritability	29.6	54.1	8.2	8.2
12	loss of interest	63.3	23.5	7.1	6.1
13	difficulty making decisions	52.0	23.5	22.4	2.0
14	feeling unattractive	65.3	20.4	11.2	3.1
15	difficulty working	19.4	41.8	29.6	9.2
16	sleep disturbance	16.3	48.0	17.3	18.4
17	tiredness	6.1	41.8	40.8	11.2
18	loss of appetite	72.4	22.4	3.1	2.0
19	weight loss	69.4	10.2	10.2	10.2
20	somatic concerns	41.8	38.8	16.3	3.1
21	loss of sexual interest	38.8	40.8	15.3	5.1

Patients were grouped according to depression scores. BDI scores of 15 or more are considered to be significant for the presence of depressive symptoms. Body mass indices did not differ in patients who had or did not have depressive symptoms (mean, 36 and 34, respectively). Similarly, ESS total scores did not differ as a function of the presence or absence of significant depressive symptoms (mean, 13.4 and 13.5, respectively). Sleep integrity, continuity, and macroarchitecture are shown in Table 3 for patients who had and did not have significant symptoms of depression. The results of statistical comparison of depression subgroup means are also included. No significant differences between groups were found for any sleep parameter. Marginal effects $(.10 > P > .05)$ were found for sleep efficiency, mean duration of the episode of rapid eye movement (REM), and REM sleep fragmentation index. Patients who did not have significant depressive symptoms tended toward lower sleep efficiencies and shorter REM sleep episodes that were less fragmented.

Discussion

The prevalence of depressive symptoms in SDB is a commonly reported phenomenon. The authors' data confirm this finding. In this patient population, the symptoms with the most extreme endorsement included (from most to least) sleep disturbance, feelings of being punished, crying, tiredness, weight loss, difficulty working, and discouragement about the future. More globally, the highest symptom endorsements were found for tiredness, sleep disturbance, difficulty working, irritability, lack of satisfaction, and loss of sexual interest. These symptoms encompass a mixture of somatic (eg, tiredness) and neurovegetative (eg, sleep disturbance) markers of depression. Symptoms of crying, feelings of being punished, and discouragement about the future are most common in melancholic depression, and it is not obvious how a sleep disturbance could produce such a profile. By contrast, sleep disturbance, irritability, and tiredness are all common symptoms of sleep disorders independent of mood instability.

In a previous study, the authors documented a strong association between SDB and psychiatric conditions [22]. The authors found that SDB confers increased risk of depression and hypothesize a possible vulnerability to mood disturbance produced by disrupted sleep and intermittent sleeplessness. In this project they focused specifically on depressive symptoms with the goal of discriminating apnea-related depression from depressed mood or dysthymia arising from other etiologies.

The authors did not find any relationship between the severity of depression and severity of apnea. The only correlation, as expected, was between sleep disruption and SaO$_2$ nadir. They found inverse relationships between symptoms related to self-esteem (feelings of failure, guilt, self disappointment, and self blame) and mean apnea duration. Longest apnea duration also correlated negatively with self blame. This profile of results ran counter to the authors' original expectations. They did not find any association between depression scores, body mass index, or sleepiness,

Table 3: **Sleep continuity, integrity, and architecture for patients with and without significant depressive symptoms (BDI > 14)**

Sleep Variable	BDI < 15		BDI > 14		
	Mean	*SD*	*Mean*	*SD*	*P*
Apnea index	20.9	19.6	21.9	25.6	ns
Apnea + hypopnea index	43.6	26.7	46.7	39.7	ns
Mean apnea duration (sec)	27.3	7.9	24.5	7.8	ns
Longest apnea episode (sec)	50.8	18.0	44.3	19.3	ns
SaO2 nadir (%)	74.2	13.9	73.6	14.2	ns
Latency to sleep (min)	9.3	14.1	9.3	12.3	ns
Sleep efficiency index	73.8	14.4	79.8	12.8	.09
Wake after sleep onset (min)	63.7	41.9	51.1	44.5	ns
Number of wakes per hour	4.5	3.0	3.6	3.4	ns
Stage 1 (% total sleep time)	14.1	10.0	11.5	11.5	ns
Stage 2 (% total sleep time)	64.4	15.6	60.6	17.1	ns
Slow-wave sleep (% total sleep time)	7.9	8.0	12.2	13.4	ns
REM Sleep % Total Sleep Time	13.5	9.8	15.8	10.5	ns
Latency to REM sleep (min)	79.8	64.2	104.6	75.0	ns
Mean REM episode duration (min)	18.7	17.2	27.6	20.0	.06
REM sleep fragmentation index	1.6	2.6	3.2	3.8	.08

although there was some evidence that patients who did not have depressive symptoms slept less efficiently. Patients who had depressive symptoms had longer mean REM sleep episodes that were more prone to fragmentation. Latency to REM sleep from sleep onset did not differ statistically between groups and was within the normal range. Furthermore, no difference between groups was found for slow-wave sleep. Thus, the common polysomnographic markers for depression were not observed in this group of subjects who had SDB; however, there was some indication of possible increased REM sleep pressure and disturbance associated with the presence of depressive symptoms.

In conclusion, depression is common in patients who have SDB, and clinicians should be alert to its presence. Patients who have SBD and high body mass indices are no more depressed than their less obese counter parts, however. Also, the degree of sleepiness is not correlated with the degree of depression. The diagnostic utility of neurovegetative symptoms such as sleep disturbances, tiredness, and weight change is poor in patients who have overlapping depression and SDB. By contrast, other symptoms would not be predicted to be shared by SDB and depression. In this population, greater emphasis for detecting primary depression should be placed on melancholic features (eg, feelings of guilt or worthlessness, self blame, ruminative thoughts, and crying). Such symptoms should be monitored after SDB treatment; if they persist, they are an indication for further evaluation and possible treatment for mood dysregulation.

References

[1] Ingram F, Henke KG, Levin HS, et al. Sleep apnea and vigilance performance in a community-dwelling older sample. Sleep 1994;17(3): 248–52.

[2] Millman RP, Fogel BS, McNamara ME, et al. Depression as a manifestation of obstructive sleep apnea: reversal with nasal continuous positive airway pressure. J Clin Psychiatry 1989;50(9): 348–51.

[3] Yue W, Hao W, Liu P, et al. A case-control study on psychological symptoms in sleep apnea-hypopnea syndrome. Can J Psychiat 2003;48: 318–23.

[4] Deldin PJ, Phillips LK, Thomas RJ. A preliminary study of sleep-disordered breathing in major depressive disorder. Sleep Med 2006;7:131–9.

[5] Sackner MA, Landa J, Forrest T, et al. Periodic sleep apnea: chronic sleep deprivation related to intermittent upper airway obstruction and central nervous system disturbance. Chest 1975; 67(2):164–71.

[6] Cheshire K, Engleman H, Deary I, et al. Factors impairing daytime performance in patients with sleep apnea/hypopnea syndrome. Arch Intern Med 1992;152(3):538–41.

[7] Jennum PJ, Sjol A. Cognitive symptoms in persons with snoring and sleep apnea. An epidemiologic study of 1.504 women and men aged 30–60 years. The Dan-MONICA II study. Ugeskr Laeger 1995;157(45):6252–6.

[8] Redline S, Strauss ME, Adams N, et al. Neuropsychological function in mild sleep disordered breathing. Sleep 1997;20(2):160–7.

[9] Coleman RM, Roffwarg HP, Kennedy SJ, et al. Sleep-wake disorders based on a polysomnographic diagnosis. A national cooperative study. JAMA 1982;247:997–1003.

[10] Flemons WW, Tsai W. Quality of life consequences of sleep-disordered breathing. J Allergy Clin Immunol 1997;99(2):S750–6.

[11] Hetzel C, Weiss HG, Schroder A, et al. Subjective well-being in obstructive sleep apnea syndrome before and after nCPAP therapy. Wien Med Wochenschr 1995;145(17–18):510–1.

[12] Derderian SS, Bridenbaugh RH, Rajagopal KR. Neuropsychologic symptoms in obstructive sleep apnea improve after treatment with nasal continuous positive airway pressure. Chest 1988;94(5):1923–7.

[13] Bosse-Henck A, Kopf A. Difficult patients in the sleep laboratory—nCPAP therapy in psychiatric patients with sleep apnea disorders. Wien Med Wochenschr 1996;146(13–14):352–4.

[14] Briones B, Adams N, Strauss M, et al. Relationship between sleepiness and general health status. Sleep 1996;19(7):583–8.

[15] Husain AM, Mebust KA, Carwile ST, et al. Depression in sleep disorders clinics. Sleep Breath 1997;2:73–5.

[16] Beck AT, Ward AC, Mendelson M, et al. An inventory for measuring depression. Arch Gen Psychiatry 1961;4:561–71.

[17] Johns MW. A new method for measuring daytime sleepiness: the Epworth Sleepiness Scale. Sleep 1991;14:540–5.

[18] Rechtschaffen A, Kales A, editors. A manual of standardized terminology, techniques and scoring system for sleep stages of human subjects. NIH Publication # 204. Washington, DC: US Government Printing Office; 1968.

[19] Bonnet M, Carley D, Carskadon M, et al. ASDA report. EEG arousals: scoring rules and examples. Sleep 1992;15:173–84.

[20] Bornstein SK. Respiratory monitoring during sleep: polysomnography. In: Guilleminault C, editor. Sleeping and waking disorders: indications and techniques. Menlo Park (CA): Addison-Wesley; 1982. p. 183–212.

[21] Bonnet M, Carley D, Guilleminault C, et al. ASDA report. Recording and scoring leg movements. Sleep 1993;16:748–59.

[22] Sharafkhaneh A, Giray N, Richardson P, et al. Association of psychiatric disorders and sleep apnea in a large cohort. Sleep 2005;28: 1405–11.

SLEEP
MEDICINE
CLINICS

Sleep Med Clin 1 (2006) 519–525

Sleep-Related Breathing Disorders and Quality of Life

Hossein Sharafkhaneh, MD[a,b,]*, Amir Sharafkhaneh, MD, D ABSM[a,b]

- Overview
- Does continuous positive airway pressure improve quality of life in patients who have obstructive sleep apnea?
- Do dental appliances improve quality of life in patients who have obstructive sleep apnea?
- Does upper airway surgery improve quality of life in patients who have obstructive sleep apnea?
- Does continuous positive airway pressure improve quality of life in patients who have obstructive sleep apnea and congestive heart failure?
- Does treatment of obstructive sleep apnea improve quality of life in children?
- Summary
- References

Overview

Sleep-related breathing disorders (SRBDs) are among the most common sleep disorders and are characterized by recurrent respiratory events. These respiratory events usually produce sleep fragmentation, hypoxia, or both. According to the International Classification of Sleep Disorders–Version 2, SRBD is one of eight major classes of sleep disorders. SRBDs include obstructive sleep apnea syndromes (OSA), central sleep apnea syndromes, sleep-related hypoventilation/hypoxemic syndromes, and "other" SRBD. According to epidemiologic studies, 4% of middle-aged men and 2% of middle-aged women have sleep apnea and excessive daytime sleepiness [1]. Age, increased body weight, increased neck circumference, and male gender are the most significant risk factors predisposing an individual to SRBD. Individuals who have SRBD commonly present with excessive daytime sleepiness, snoring, morning headache, fatigue, daytime naps, witnessed apneas, and falling asleep while driving. SRBD is associated with systemic hypertension, myocardial infarction, heart failure, cardiac dysrhythmias, stroke, neurocognitive dysfunction, personality changes, motor vehicle and industrial accidents, and impaired quality of life (QOL) [2–4].

Chronic medical and psychiatric conditions adversely affect the individual's daytime functioning and ability to perform activities of daily living. OSA is a chronic condition that gradually impairs the individual's ability to function and thereby impairs QOL. Increasingly, more attention is being paid to evaluation of SRBD's contribution to diminished QOL [5]. QOL is assessed using self-administered questionnaires. These instruments are intended to evaluate the effect of a disease and its treatment on the patient from his or her point of view. Table 1 shows frequently used questionnaires

[a] Sleep Disorders & Research Center, Michael E. DeBakey Veterans Affairs Medical Center, 2002 Holcombe Blvd., Houston, TX 77030, USA
[b] Baylor College of Medicine, 1 Baylor Plaza, Houston, TX 77030, USA
* Corresponding author. Sleep Center (111i), 2002 Holcombe Blvd., Houston, TX 77030.
E-mail address: hosseins@bcm.tmc.edu (H. Sharafkhaneh).

Table 1: **Frequently used quality-of-life questionnaires and their domains**

Questionnaire (Complete Name)	Type	Domains
Medical Outcome Survey Short Form-36 (SF-36)	Generic	Physical role Vitality Social functioning Mental health Bodily pain Physical functioning Emotional role General health
Calgary Sleep Apnea Quality of Life Instrument (SAQLI)	Specific	Daily functioning Social interactions Emotional functioning Symptoms
Obstructive Sleep Disorders-6 survey (OSD-6)	Specific	Physical suffering Sleep disturbance Speech and swallowing difficulties Emotional distress Activity limitation Level of concern of the caregiver associated with the patient's illness and related symptoms
Functional Outcomes of Sleep Questionnaire (FOSQ)	Specific	General productivity Social outcome Activity level Vigilance Intimacy and sexual relationships
Franco's Pediatric Obstructive Sleep Apnea instrument (OSA-18)	Specific	Sleep disturbance Physical suffering Emotional distress Daytime problems Caregiver concerns

for QOL assessment in patients who have OSA. There are two types of questionnaires: generic and specific [6]. Generic questionnaires are designed to evaluate QOL in patients who have a range of chronic disorders. Specific questionnaires are designed to evaluate particular aspects of life that are affected by a given condition or disease (eg, OSA). Therefore the generic tools are applicable in multiple chronic disorders, whereas the specific tools are applicable only for the target disease for which they were developed. The Medical Outcome Survey Short Form-36 (SF-36) is an example of a generic instrument; the Functional Outcomes of Sleep Questionnaire (FOSQ) and Calgary Sleep Apnea Quality of Life Instrument (SAQLI) are examples of disease-specific instruments [7,8]. Each QOL questionnaire has assorted domains; in each domain several questions evaluate some more or less focused aspect of QOL. Early studies reported significantly diminished QOL in patients who had moderate-to-severe OSA and robust improvement with continuous positive airway pressure (CPAP) therapy. The effect of CPAP in patients who have mild OSA is less clear. This article briefly reviews recent publications that evaluated effects of OSA treatment on QOL.

Does continuous positive airway pressure improve quality of life in patients who have obstructive sleep apnea?

Generic and specific QOL tools show a worsening of QOL with OSA and improvement in with treatment. West and colleagues [9] randomly assigned 98 patients who had OSA to three different groups. Patients in group one underwent 6 months of auto-titration, patients in group two underwent 1 week of auto-titration followed by CPAP for 6 months, and patients in group three underwent fixed-pressure treatment based on neck size and dip rate [9]. The authors measured QOL with the SF-36 and SAQLI at baseline and after 1 and 6 months of intervention. QOL improved significantly on all scores and in all groups following treatment. No significant differences were found between groups on any of the measured outcomes.

In a randomized, controlled clinical trial, Mador and coworkers [10] studied 98 patients who had polysomnographically diagnosed OSA. Patients were divided into two groups. In group one, 49 patients were assigned to CPAP (control). In group two, 49 patients were assigned to CPAP plus heated humidifier. There were no significant differences between the two groups in mean apnea-hypopnea index (AHI), mean age, and mean Epworth Sleepiness Scale (ESS). QOL was evaluated using the SAQLI at baseline, 1 month, 3 months, and after 12 months of using CPAP, with or without heated humidification. QOL improved in both groups but did not differ significantly between the two groups. In another randomized, parallel-designed study, 91 patients suffering from severe OSA were randomly assigned to two groups. The 51 patients in group one used CPAP with pressure set according to body mass index for the first 3 months followed by standard titrated CPAP for the second 3 months. By contrast, the 40 patients in group two used standard CPAP for 3 months [11]. There were no significant differences between groups for age and AHI. QOL improved in both groups. The SF-36 scores for the vitality, role-emotional, and mental health domains improved across both treatment groups. By contrast, the general health domain improved only in the arbitrary-pressure arm. In a complementary way, social functioning improved significantly in the study-determined CPAP pressure arm [11].

Whitelaw and colleagues [12] studied 288 subjects with prior diagnostic polysomnography in a randomized clinical 4-week trial of auto-titration versus home oximetry. QOL was evaluated using the SF-36 and SAQLI at baseline and after 4 weeks of treatment. QOL improved with no significant difference between study arms in various domains of the SF-36, although there were higher mean increases in the SAQLI in the polysomnography group than in the home-monitoring group.

Thirty-one patients who had mild sleep apnea (mean AHI, 21.6) participated in a randomized, controlled, crossover clinical trial [13]. QOL was assessed with the SF-36 and FOSQ, and no significant QOL improvements were found between standard CPAP and sham CPAP. Sleepiness improved significantly, however.

In short-term, randomized, clinical trial, Senn and colleagues [14] used the SF-36 to evaluate 29 patients who had severe OSA (mean AHI, 46 ± 4) at baseline and after 3 months of using CPAP. The subjects were assigned randomly to an auto-CPAP device responding to apnea–hypopnea and snoring in group one, to an auto-CPAP device responding to snoring and changes in flow contour in group two, and to fixed CPAP set to the 90th pressure percentile titrated by auto-CPAP over 2 weeks in group three. They found significant improvements in SF-36 health transition, vitality, and social functioning

scores and in the mental component summary scores in all treatment modalities and no change in other domains of the SF-36 questionnaire. They concluded that both auto-CPAP devices were as effective as fixed-pressure CPAP for improving QOL. In another randomized trial, which used a crossover design, 39 patients were evaluated with the FOSQ at baseline and at 3 and 6 weeks after using CPAP with nasal pillows (group one) and CPAP with a nasal mask (group two) [15]. Study investigators found significant improvement in the total FOSQ score in both groups and no differences between two groups in FOSQ total score or any of the domains. Still another randomized, placebo-controlled trial evaluated the effect of 1 week of CPAP versus placebo on 39 patients diagnosed as having OSA [16]. Patients were assessed with the SF-36 at baseline and after intervention. In this study, several aspects of QOL improved in both groups over time with no difference between the two groups. The investigators also found significant time effects for the following subscales of the Medical Outcomes Survey: satisfaction with physical functioning, effects of pain, pain severity, cognitive functioning, mental health index I, psychologic well-being I, depression/behavioral-emotional control, anxiety I, psychologic distress I, positive affect II, mental health index II, psychologic distress II, anxiety II, psychologic well-being II, mental health index III, role limitations cause by emotional problems, and physical/physiologic functioning. Notably, these changes over time were observed in both groups.

To determine QOL changes in patients who had mild sleep apnea (AHI = 12.9; ESS = 11; n = 28), an 8-week randomized, placebo-controlled, crossover clinical trial compared CPAP with placebo tablet. After CPAP was used, all domains of FOSQ improved except for intimate relationship and sexual activity [17]. Further, there was a placebo effect in all domains except for general productivity. In the SF-36, authors reported significant placebo effect on patient perception of physical functioning, role limitations caused by emotional problems, mental health, and energy/vitality. There was improvement in three of the eight domains (social functioning, mental health, and energy/vitality), but in no area was there a significant difference between the improvement seen with CPAP and that with placebo.

Thus the literature overwhelmingly supports the notion that CPAP therapy of OSA improves QOL in moderate-to-severe chronic obstructive pulmonary disease. In milder forms of OSA, however, the studies are less clear, perhaps because daily life is less severely impaired in mild OSA. In addition, the likelihood of a therapeutic adherence with the treatment is less in patients who have mild OSA, especially if they are not sleepy.

Do dental appliances improve quality of life in patients who have obstructive sleep apnea?

Dental appliances that advance the mandible are effective in lowering the AHI. The devices are recommended mostly for treating mild-to-moderate OSA. In contrast, these devices are not recommended as first-line therapy for severe OSA or breathing disorders associated with prominent oxygen desaturations. CPAP generally is regarded as more effective than dental appliances in lowering AHI; however, published studies report that patients prefer the dental appliances [18].

Barnes and colleagues [19] used the SF-36 and FOSQ in a randomized, controlled, three-way crossover trial to evaluate 114 patients at baseline and after 3 months of intervention. These patients had OSA according to overnight polysomnography. The interventions were CPAP therapy, mandibular advancement splint, and placebo tablet. Compared with placebo, mandibular advancement splint treatment improved QOL as measured by the FOSQ mean score and social outcome domain and by the SF-36 overall health score. CPAP treatment was effective with respect to FOSQ overall score and activity level, as well as the SF-36 mean score and well-being. In a randomized trial, Walker-Engstrom and colleagues [20] evaluated change in QOL using the Minor Symptoms Evaluation-Profile after treatment with a dental appliance or uvulopalatopharyngoplasty in 95 patients who had mild-to-moderate OSA. Both groups showed significant improvement in QOL. In summary, dental appliances improve QOL in mild-to-moderate forms of OSA.

Does upper airway surgery improve quality of life in patients who have obstructive sleep apnea?

Although CPAP is the treatment of choice for OSA, surgery may be indicated to treat OSA in patients in whom an underlying specific, surgically correctable abnormality causes the sleep apnea [21]. In addition, surgery may be indicated to treat OSA in patients for whom other noninvasive treatments have been unsuccessful or have been rejected, who desire surgery, and who are medically stable enough to undergo the procedure.

In a clinical trial, Lin and colleagues [22] studied 139 subjects suffering from moderate-to-severe OSA. Eighty-four subjects used CPAP machine, and 55 subjects underwent extended uvulopalatoplasty (EUPF). These patients were evaluated by the Snore Outcome Survey and SF-36 at baseline, 6 months, and 3 years after intervention. The study showed that EUPF had a better effect on snoring than CPAP 6 months after intervention. This effect gradually declined at the 3-year follow-up examination. Further, improvements in the QOL with EUPF were equal to those with CPAP treatment. In the CPAP group five of the eight SF-36 subscale scores (physical functioning, general health, vitality, social functioning, and mental health) were improved significantly after 6 months, and the effect was maintained until the 3-year follow-up. Seven of the eight SF-36 subscale scores were improved significantly immediately after EUPF, and the effect persisted for 3 years. (The exception was general health.) Finally, there was no significant difference in the improvement in SF-36 scores between the CPAP and surgery groups.

Woodson and colleagues [23], in a randomized, placebo-controlled clinical trial, evaluated the effect of temperature-controlled radio frequency tissue ablation (TCRFTA) versus CPAP and sham placebo on QOL in 87 patients who had mild OSA. QOL was evaluated with the SF-36 and FOSQ at baseline and 8 weeks after intervention. The authors reported that QOL improved with TCRFTA and CPAP compared with sham placebo. The two active-intervention arms did not differ in regard to measured outcomes. In summary, upper airway surgery aiming at reducing the obstruction improves QOL when it diminishes the AHI.

Does continuous positive airway pressure improve quality of life in patients who have obstructive sleep apnea and congestive heart failure?

Heart failure is one of the leading causes of morbidity and mortality in the United States. More than 5 million patients in the United States suffer from heart failure, with nearly 500,000 cases diagnosed each year [24]. Approximately 300,000 patients die yearly of heart failure. Despite recent advances in management of heart failure, the number of deaths has increased steadily [24,25]. Sleep-disordered breathing is prevalent in patients who have heart failure. Multiple studies reveal a strong association between systolic cardiac dysfunction and the occurrence of SRBD. At least 45% of patients who have heart failure have an AHI. Javaheri and colleagues [26] reported that 51% of 81 subjects who had an ejection fraction of less than 45% and clinically stable heart failure had an AHI. The subgroup that had sleep-disordered breathing had more sleep fragmentation, more severe hypoxia, stayed longer in O_2 saturation below 90%, and had less rapid-eye-movement sleep. Central sleep apnea is more frequent than OSA in patients who have systolic heart failure [27,28]. In patients who have systolic heart failure the presence of sleep-disordered breathing is associated with poor outcome. Patients who have systolic heart failure and sleep-disordered breathing are more limited in their physical performance [29], develop dyspnea at lower work loads [29], have more cardiac arrhythmia [26], have more complex arrhythmias [30], and have higher mortality than patients who have heart failure but do not have sleep-disordered breathing [31–34]. Lanfranchi [35] found that the AHI, independent of other risk factors, is a powerful predictor of poor prognosis.

Several studies reported improved sleep quality and daytime cardiac function with CPAP therapy in patients who have OSA [36]. In a randomized, controlled clinical trial, 55 patients suffering from congestive heart failure and OSA were evaluated by the SF-36 and Chronic Heart Failure Questionnaire (a disease-specific QOL instrument) at baseline and after 3 months [37]. The study participants were assigned randomly to two groups. The 29 patients in group one (mean age, 57.2 + 1.7 years; mean AHI, 28.3 + 0.4; ESS, 10.7 + 0.7) used CPAP for 3 months. The 27 patients in group two, the control group (mean age, 57.5 + 1.6 years; mean AHI, 28.1 + 3.9; ESS, 9.2 + 0.9), did not use CPAP during that period. Nineteen patients in group one and 21 patients in group two were able to complete the study. Investigators found improvements in the eight domains of the SF-36 questionnaire, especially in the domains of physical role, social functioning, and mental health. Further, significant improvements in three of four domains (fatigue, emotional well-being, and disease mastery) of the chronic heart failure questionnaire were reported; the dyspnea domain did not change significantly. The result of CPAP therapy on QOL in this group of patients who had OSA and congestive heart failure was similar to that in patients who had OSA but did not have congestive heart failure.

Does treatment of obstructive sleep apnea improve quality of life in children?

OSA caused by adenotonsillar hypertrophy or obesity is an increasing problem in children [38]. The literature indicates a strong association between OSA and poor performance and attention deficit disorder in the pediatric population [39]. Mitchell and associates [40] performed a clinical trial in 60 children (mean age, 7.1 years) suffering from OSA (mean AHI, 28). Patients were evaluated by the Obstructive Sleep Apnea-18 (a QOL questionnaire) at baseline and within 6 months of surgery (adenotonsillectomy). The authors concluded that the total Obstructive Sleep Apnea-18 score, the scores for all domains, and scores for all items showed significant improvement after surgery. A decrease in the Obstructive Sleep Apnea-18 total score greater than 20 points was noted in 48 children (80%), and a decrease greater than 10 points was noted in 51 children (85%).

Diez-Montiel and colleagues [41], in a controlled, clinical trial, evaluated 101 children using the Obstructive Sleep Disorders-6 survey, a validated tool for assessing QOL in children who have OSA, at three points: before surgery (adenoidectomy alone, tonsillectomy alone, or adenotonsillectomy), 8 days after the surgery, and 36 to 75 months after the surgery. Patients were diagnosed as having OSA based on the history, physical examination, radiographic films of the lateral aspect of the neck, and overnight pulse oximetry. Pulse oximetry was considered positive when the patient had two or more episodes of desaturation under 90%. The study showed a significant improvement in all six domains with treatment. These two studies clearly showed that treatment of OSA in pediatric patients improves QOL.

Summary

OSA diminishes QOL. The clinical literature overwhelmingly indicates improvement in QOL with adequate treatment of OSA. The effect on QOL is seen regardless of (1) type of treatment and (2) presence of underlying comorbid cardiovascular disease. Improvement is seen quickly, in as little as 4 weeks after initiation of treatment. The literature also shows similar effects on QOL in pediatric OSA. Further studies are needed to evaluate long-term effects of OSA therapy on QOL. Specifically, it is not clearly known if the surgical interventions, fixed-pressure CPAP, or use of a dental appliance will maintain their efficacy over time, especially as patients age or gain weight.

References

[1] Young T, Palta M, Dempsey J, et al. The occurrence of sleep-disordered breathing among middle-aged adults. N Engl J Med 1993;328(17):1230–5.

[2] Chervin RD, Guilleminault C. Obstructive sleep apnea and related disorders. Neurol Clin 1996;14(3):583–609.

[3] Tilkian AG, Guilleminault C, Schroeder JS, et al. Sleep-induced apnea syndrome. Prevalence of cardiac arrhythmias and their reversal after tracheostomy. Am J Med 1977;63(3):348–58.

[4] Peppard PE, Young T, Palta M, et al. Prospective study of the association between sleep-disordered

breathing and hypertension. N Engl J Med 2000; 342(19):1378–84.

[5] Weaver TE. Outcome measurement in sleep medicine practice and research. Part 1: assessment of symptoms, subjective and objective daytime sleepiness, health-related quality of life and functional status. Sleep Med Rev 2001;5(2):103–28.

[6] Moyer CA, Sonnad SS, Garetz SL, et al. Quality of life in obstructive sleep apnea: a systematic review of the literature. Sleep Med 2001;2(6):477–91.

[7] Weaver TE, Laizner AM, Evans LK, et al. An instrument to measure functional status outcomes for disorders of excessive sleepiness. Sleep 1997; 20(10):835–43.

[8] Flemons WW, Reimer MA. Development of a disease-specific health-related quality of life questionnaire for sleep apnea. Am J Respir Crit Care Med 1998;158(2):494–503.

[9] West SD, Jones DR, Stradling JR. Comparison of three ways to determine and deliver pressure during nasal CPAP therapy for obstructive sleep apnoea. Thorax 2006;61(3):226–31.

[10] Mador MJ, Krauza M, Pervez A, et al. Effect of heated humidification on compliance and quality of life in patients with sleep apnea using nasal continuous positive airway pressure. Chest 2005; 128(4):2151–8.

[11] Hukins CA. Arbitrary-pressure continuous positive airway pressure for obstructive sleep apnea syndrome. Am J Respir Crit Care Med 2005; 171(5):500–5.

[12] Whitelaw WA, Brant RF, Flemons WW. Clinical usefulness of home oximetry compared with polysomnography for assessment of sleep apnea. Am J Respir Crit Care Med 2005;171(2): 188–93.

[13] Marshall NS, Neill AM, Campbell AJ, et al. Randomised controlled crossover trial of humidified continuous positive airway pressure in mild obstructive sleep apnoea. Thorax 2005;60(5):427–32.

[14] Senn O, Brack T, Matthews F, et al. Randomized short-term trial of two AutoCPAP devices versus fixed continuous positive airway pressure for the treatment of sleep apnea. Am J Respir Crit Care Med 2003;168(12):1506–11.

[15] Massie CA, Hart RW. Clinical outcomes related to interface type in patients with obstructive sleep apnea/hypopnea syndrome who are using continuous positive airway pressure. Chest 2003;123(4):1112–8.

[16] Profant J, Ancoli-Israel S, Dimsdale JEA. Randomized, controlled trial of 1 week of continuous positive airway pressure treatment on quality of Life. Heart Lung 2003;32(1):52–8.

[17] Barnes M, Houston D, Worsnop CJ, et al. A randomized controlled trial of continuous positive airway pressure in mild obstructive sleep apnea. Am J Respir Crit Care Med 2002;165(6):773–80.

[18] Ferguson KA, Lowe AA. Oral appliances for sleep-disordered breathing. In: Kryger M, Roth T, Dement WC, editors. Principles and practice of sleep medicine. 4th edition. Philadelphia: Elsevier Saunders; 2005. p. 1098–108.

[19] Barnes M, McEvoy RD, Banks S, et al. Efficacy of positive airway pressure and oral appliance in mild to moderate obstructive sleep apnea. Am J Respir Crit Care Med 2004;170(6):656–64.

[20] Walker-Engstrom ML, Wilhelmsson B, Tegelberg A, et al. Quality of life assessment of treatment with dental appliance or UPPP in patients with mild to moderate obstructive sleep apnoea. A prospective randomized 1-year follow-up study. J Sleep Res 2000;9(3):303–8.

[21] Thorpy M, Chesson A, Derderian S, et al. Practice parameters for the treatment of obstructive sleep apnea in adults: the efficacy of surgical modifications of the upper airway. Sleep 1996; 19:152–5.

[22] Lin SW, Chen NH, Li HY, et al. A comparison of the long-term outcome and effects of surgery or continuous positive airway pressure on patients with obstructive sleep apnea syndrome. Laryngoscope 2006;116(6):1012–6.

[23] Woodson BT, Steward DL, Weaver EM, et al. A randomized trial of temperature-controlled radiofrequency, continuous positive airway pressure, and placebo for obstructive sleep apnea syndrome. Otolaryngol Head Neck Surg 2003; 128(6):848–61.

[24] American College of Cardiology/American Heart Association practice guidelines. ACC/AHA guideline for management of the evaluation and management of chronic heart failure. Circulation 2001;104:2996–3007.

[25] Bradley TD, Floras JS. Sleep apnea and heart failure: part i: obstructive sleep apnea. Circulation 2003;107(12):1671–8.

[26] Javaheri S, Parker TJ, Liming JD, et al. Sleep apnea in 81 ambulatory male patients with stable heart failure. Types and their prevalences, consequences, and presentations. Circulation 1998; 97(21):2154–9.

[27] Sin DD, Fitzgerald F, Parker JD, et al. Risk factors for central and obstructive sleep apnea in 450 men and women with congestive heart failure. Am J Respir Crit Care Med 1999; 160(4):1101–6.

[28] Tremel F, Pepin JL, Veale D, et al. High prevalence and persistence of sleep apnoea in patients referred for acute left ventricular failure and medically treated over 2 months. Eur Heart J 1999;20(16):1201–9.

[29] Wright DJ, Tan LB. The role of exercise testing in the evaluation and management of heart failure. Postgrad Med J 1999;75(886):453–8.

[30] Massumi RA, Nutter DO. Cardiac arrhythmias associated with Cheyne-Stokes respiration: a note on the possible mechanisms. Dis Chest 1968;54(1):21–32.

[31] Ancoli-Israel S, DuHamel ER, Stepnowsky C, et al. The relationship between congestive heart failure, sleep apnea, and mortality in older men. Chest 2003;124(4):1400–5.

[32] Andreas S, Hagenah G, Moller C, et al. Cheyne-Stokes respiration and prognosis in congestive heart failure. Am J Cardiol. 12–1-1996;78(11):1260–4.

[33] Hanly PJ, Zuberi-Khokhar NS. Increased mortality associated with Cheyne-Stokes respiration in patients with congestive heart failure. Am J Respir Crit Care Med 1996;153(1):272–6.

[34] Wilcox I, McNamara SG, Wessendorf T, et al. Prognosis and sleep disordered breathing in heart failure. Thorax 1998;53(Suppl 3):S33–6.

[35] Lanfranchi PA, Braghiroli A, Bosimini E, et al. Prognostic value of nocturnal Cheyne-Stokes respiration in chronic heart failure. Circulation 1999;99(11):1435–40.

[36] Arzt M, Bradley TD. Treatment of sleep apnea in heart failure. Am J Respir Crit Care Med 2006; 173(12):1300–8.

[37] Mansfield DR, Gollogly NC, Kaye DM, et al. Controlled trial of continuous positive airway pressure in obstructive sleep apnea and heart failure. Am J Respir Crit Care Med 2004; 169(3):361–6.

[38] Ng DK, Chan C, Chow AS, et al. Childhood sleep-disordered breathing and its implications for cardiac and vascular diseases. J Paediatr Child Health 2005;41(12):640–6.

[39] Kheirandish L, Gozal D. Neurocognitive dysfunction in children with sleep disorders. Dev Sci 2006;9(4):388–99.

[40] Mitchell RB, Kelly J, Call E, et al. Quality of Life after adenotonsillectomy for obstructive sleep apnea in children. Arch Otolaryngol Head Neck Surg 2004;130(2):190–4.

[41] Diez-Montiel A, de Diego JI, Prim MP, et al. Quality of life after surgical treatment of children with obstructive sleep apnea: long-term results. Int J Pediatr Otorhinolaryngol 2006;70(9): 1575–9.

SLEEP
MEDICINE
CLINICS

Sleep Med Clin 1 (2006) 527–531

Positive Airway Pressure Therapy for Obstructive Sleep Apnea

Teofilo Lee-Chiong, MD[a],*, Max Hirshkowitz, PhD, D ABSM[b,c]

- Indications for positive airway pressure therapy
- Adequacy of positive airway pressure titration in obstructive sleep apnea
  - *Optimal titration*
  - *Good titration*
  - *Adequate titration*
- *Unacceptable titration*
- Benefits of positive airway pressure therapy
- Therapeutic adherence
- Autotitrating positive airway pressure
- Summary
- References

For most patients who have obstructive sleep apnea (OSA), positive airway pressure is the treatment of choice. It consists of a fan or turbine-driven flow generator, a connecting tube, and a patient interface. The patient interface is usually a nasal mask; however, it can be a nasal-oral mask, an oral mask, or nasal pillows. The flow generator provides a positive pressure designed to counteract the negative intrathoracic pressure during inhalation that collapses the airway. The positive pressure creates a pneumatic splint and thereby maintains airway patency. There are essentially three types of positive pressure devices currently available for treating obstructive sleep apnea.

The positive pressure can be continuous and fixed at a set pressure. This is the most common form and is called continuous positive airway pressure (CPAP). Its use in treating OSA was described initially by Sullivan and colleagues [1] in 1981. In their report, five patients who had severe OSA were treated with CPAP applied through the nares. Low pressure levels (ranging from 4.5–10 cm H_2O)

completely prevented upper airway occlusion, allowing uninterrupted sleep.

By contrast, the positive pressure device can have two settings and switch automatically between a higher pressure during inspiration and a lower pressure during expiration. Such devices are designated bilevel positive airway pressure (BPAP). The pressure drop during exhalation may increase comfort for patients who have trouble exhaling against an incoming pressure. A variant of BPAP was developed to offer ventilatory assistance. It is similar to BPAP, but it paces the two different pressures at a set rate to entrain breathing. Devices of this design provide noninvasive positive pressure ventilation.

Finally, a third type of positive pressure device generates variable flow. Flow is controlled by computer algorithms designed to seek continually an optimal pressure. These autotitrating positive airway pressure (APAP) devices constantly readjust pressures in response to changing physiologic and functional requirements.

[a] National Jewish Medical and Research Center, J232 1400 Jackson Street, Denver, CO 80206, USA
[b] Sleep Disorders & Research Center, Michael E. DeBakey Veterans Affairs Medical Center, 2002 Holcombe Blvd., Houston, TX 77030, USA
[c] Baylor College of Medicine, 1 Baylor Plaza, Houston, TX 77030, USA
* Corresponding author.
E-mail address: max8@bmc.tmc.edu (T. Lee-Chiong).

1556-407X/06/$ – see front matter © 2006 Elsevier Inc. All rights reserved.
sleep.theclinics.com

doi:10.1016/j.jsmc.2006.11.002

To be optimally effective, the positive pressure level must be titrated. Titration allows the clinician to select proper pressures. CPAP and BPAP usually are titrated during an overnight, laboratory-based, polysomnography. APAP is designed to self-titrate at home or in the laboratory. Several methods have been proposed for pressure selection (Table 1). The goal of each procedure is to eliminate apnea, hypopnea, snoring, and respiratory effort–related arousals in all body positions and sleep stages. Higher pressures often are required to prevent airway occlusion during rapid eye movement (REM) sleep than during nonREM sleep, except in patients who have heart failure. Additionally, sleep-disordered breathing is usually worse when an individual sleeps supine.

Indications for positive airway pressure therapy

There is not complete agreement concerning the criteria for treatment with positive airway pressure. Different agencies and insurance carriers have different minimum criteria for prescribing positive airway pressure. Nonetheless, diagnostic criteria for prescribing positive airway pressure therapy usually is based on sleep evaluations using attended, laboratory polysomnography. Table 2 shows treatment criteria for positive airway pressure prescriptions according to guidelines set forth by the American Academy of Sleep Medicine [2] and Medicare [3].

Adequacy of positive airway pressure titration in obstructive sleep apnea

In rating positive airway pressure titration, the goal is to eliminate sleep pathophysiology. Sometimes it is not possible to achieve the goal; however, the night technologist does the best he or she can. The following grading scheme was developed at the authors' center to provide information about the adequacy of positive airway pressure titrations and to help track therapeutic intervention.

Optimal titration

An optimal titration reduces the respiratory distress index (RDI) to fewer than five events per hour of sleep. This level of reduction often is difficult to achieve. The interval during which the chosen pressure is administered must contain at least 15 minutes of sleep, contain some REM sleep, and not be continually interrupted by arousals or awakenings.

Good titration

In patients who have moderate-to-severe sleep-related breathing disorder (SRBD) (apnea index or RDI > 20), a good titration must reduce RDI to 10 or less. Indices at this level are considered within the normal range. By contrast, in patients who have mild SRBD with a baseline RDI of less than 20, a good titration must reduce RDI by 50% or more. The interval during which the chosen pressure is administered must contain at least 15 minutes of sleep, contain some REM sleep, and not be continually interrupted by arousals or awakenings.

Adequate titration

In patients for whom normal values (RDI ≤ 10) are not achieved even though sleep-related breathing is greatly improved, an adequate titration is one that

Table 1: Positive pressure selection procedures

Procedure name	Procedure description
Full-night	Technologist manually adjusts the pressure during an attended, all-night, laboratory polysomnographic recording attempting to eliminate all or most of the obstructive respiratory events.
Split-night	After an initial ≥ 2 hours of polysomnographic recording used to diagnose obstructive sleep apnea, the technologist applies the mask. Once the patient is comfortable with the mask, the technologist begins manually adjusting pressure until all or most of the obstructive respiratory events are eliminated. Calculation: Sleep specialist uses formula to derive pressures from clinical, polysomnographic, and/or anthropometric variables. The calculated pressure can also be used as a starting CPAP pressure for laboratory titration.
Autotitration	Unattended home or laboratory recordings using autotitrating devices.

Abbreviation: CPAP, continuous positive airway pressure.

Table 2: Indications for using positive airway pressure			
Criteria	Patient characteristics	Full-night	Split-night
American Academy of Sleep Medicine	Asymptomatic patients	RDI ≥ 15	AHI ≥ 40
	Patients who have excessive daytime sleepiness	RDI ≥ 5	AHI ≥ 20
Medicare	Asymptomatic patients	AHI > 15	AHI > 15
	Patients who have comorbidities[a]	AHI > 5	AHI > 5

Abbreviations: AHI, apnea plus hypopnea index; RDI, respiratory disturbance index.
[a] Comorbidities include impaired cognition, mood disorder, insomnia, hypertension, heart disease, and stroke.

reduces RDI by 75% or more. Such patients should be followed closely clinically with a re-evaluation as needed. Another reason for a titration being adequate rather than good or optimal is that REM sleep did not occur during the best pressure. This circumstance can arise because of medication-related REM suppression, inadequate REM sleep during the sleep evaluation, insufficient time for REM to occur late in the night, and satiation of REM sleep drive because of rebound earlier in the study. In such cases, the sleep specialist must rely on clinical judgment and should document the basis for deciding about titration adequacy. Such patients should be followed closely clinically with a re-evaluation, as needed.

Unacceptable titration

An unacceptable titration is one that fails to meet even minimally adequate titration criteria. The patient should be re-evaluated, or other treatment options should be applied. Sometimes an estimated positive airway pressure level can be based on a clear-cut and substantial reduction in SRBD events. If an estimate is made, there should be close follow-up with a retitration if symptoms (including but not limited to snoring, daytime somnolence, and observed apneas during sleep) do not resolve.

Benefits of positive airway pressure therapy

Positive airway pressure therapy is both safe and effective. It can be used in patients who have mild, moderate, or severe SRBD. Sleepiness decreases, alertness improves, and overall quality of life increases in response to positive airway pressure therapy in patients who have sleep-disordered breathing [4]. Decreases in sleepiness and other OSA-related clinical symptoms and improvements in quality of life in patients receiving CPAP and conservative therapy (sleep hygiene and weight loss) compare better with those seen in patients receiving only conservative therapy [5,6]. Additionally, for patients who adhere to recommended CPAP use, a significant reduction in health care use (physician claims and hospitalizations) were documented 2 years after diagnosis and treatment of OSA [7].

Lavie and colleagues [8] observed a linear increase in blood pressure and number of patients with hypertension as a function of sleep apnea severity (based on the apnea plus hypopnea index) [9–11]. In the classic study by He and colleagues [12], increased mortality was found in association with sleep-disordered breathing. In a sample of 385 men who had OSA, greater mortality occurred in those who had 20 or more apneas per hour of sleep than in those who had fewer apneic events. This difference in apnea-associated mortality was more evident in younger patients (age < 50 years), in whom all-cause mortality is less frequent.

Therapeutic adherence

CPAP therapy is only as beneficial as its use. Thus, less-than-optimal CPAP use is a significant problem in clinical practice. To a large extent, the level of use has as much to do with the individual as it does with the therapy. Although a noticeably beneficial therapy may lead to somewhat greater adherence in willing patients, a noxious intervention can discourage use in even the most ardent and willing participant. Therefore, correcting mask problems, discomfort, nasal allergies, and other barriers to use, especially during the first few months, is critical to achieve therapeutic adherence. The first month of therapy also predicts later use because it provides a baseline for how much an individual is likely to accept any therapy or be discouraged by its associated difficulties. Marketing theory predicts greatest sales (or use) in those who believe a product is beneficial and also believe that they can change their behavior to use the product. Any doubt about the product's usefulness or about one's ability to use the product acts as a barrier to use.

Autotitrating positive airway pressure

The pressure needed to maintain airway patency may vary significantly over the course of a single night. Sleep-stage variations associated with changes in body position frequently produce differing pressure requirements [2,13]. Additionally, night-to-night variability can be provoked by a host of factors. APAP can be a useful tool for the clinic as well as therapy for the patient. In one study, 49.3% of home treatment time on APAP was spent at a pressure equal to or less than the effective pressure level determined during a polysomnographic recording [14]. Higher pressures increase the propensity of mask leaks, mouth leaks, and pressure intolerance. Another application of APAP technology involves using the device to identify a fixed single pressure for subsequent treatment with a conventional CPAP device (APAP titration). Several studies have compared APAP titration with conventional CPAP titration.

Autoadjusting APAP compares favorably with CPAP. Twenty-five patients who had OSA randomly assigned to treatment with APAP and then CPAP, or vice versa, did not differ in apnea-hypopnea index, awakening/arousal index, slow-wave sleep duration, nocturnal oxygen saturation, self-reported sleepiness, or nightly usage. The mean pressure required was significantly lower with APAP than with CPAP [15]. Similar results were found in other studies [16]. Substituting APAP titration for conventional CPAP titration was studied in 122 patients during their titration night. Subsequent acceptance of CPAP by patients was not affected by APAP titration compared with conventional CPAP titration: 73% of patients who had APAP titration and 64% of those who had CPAP titration were successfully established on CPAP at week 6 [17]. APAP devices currently are not recommended for split-night studies.

Summary

Positive airway pressure is the preferred treatment for OSA. Positive pressure devices come in three varieties, of which CPAP is the most commonly prescribed. Positive airway pressure creates airway patency during sleep, leading to improved sleep quality, sleep continuity, daytime alertness, and overall quality of life in symptomatic patients who have moderate or severe OSA. Further studies are needed to assess the benefits of CPAP therapy for patients who have less-severe OSA and to specify better the positive cardiovascular outcomes. The effectiveness of CPAP is compromised because a large proportion of patients cannot tolerate or do not regularly use the mask and machine.

APAP holds great promise but at present is not recommended as a replacement for laboratory titration. Overall, positive airway pressure is a safe and effective treatment for patients who have SRBD.

References

[1] Sullivan CE, Issa FG, Berthon-Jones M, et al. Reversal of obstructive sleep apnoea by continuous positive airway pressure applied through the nares. Lancet 1981;1(8225):862–5.

[2] Standards of Practice Committee of the American Academy of Sleep Medicine. Practice parameters for the use of auto-titrating continuous positive airway pressure devices for titrating pressures and treating adult patients with obstructive sleep apnea syndrome. An American Academy of Sleep Medicine Report. Sleep 2002;25(2):143–7.

[3] Raj R, Hirshkowitz M. Effect of the new Medicare guideline on patient qualification for positive airway pressure therapy. Sleep Med 2003;4:29–33.

[4] Jenkinson C, Davies RJ, Mullins R, et al. Comparison of therapeutic and subtherapeutic nasal continuous positive airway pressure for obstructive sleep apnoea: a randomised prospective parallel trial. Lancet 1999;353(9170):2100–5.

[5] Engleman HM, Martin SE, Deary IJ, et al. Effect of CPAP therapy on daytime function in patients with mild sleep apnoea/hypopnoea syndrome. Thorax 1997;52(2):114–9.

[6] Engleman HM, Kingshott RN, Wraith PK, et al. Randomized placebo-controlled crossover trial of continuous positive airway pressure for mild sleep apnea/hypopnea syndrome. Am J Respir Crit Care Med 1999;159(2):461.

[7] Bahammam A, Delaive K, Ronald J, et al. Health care utilization in males with obstructive sleep apnea syndrome two years after diagnosis and treatment. Sleep 1999;22(6):740–7.

[8] Lavie P, Herer P, Hoffstein V. Obstructive sleep apnoea syndrome as a risk factor for hypertension: population study. BMJ 2000;320(7233):479–82.

[9] Suzuki M, Otsuka K, Guilleminault C. Long-term nasal continuous positive airway pressure administration can normalize hypertension in obstructive sleep apnea patients. Sleep 1993;16(6):545–9.

[10] Faccenda JF, Mackay TW, Boon NA, et al. Randomized placebo-controlled trial of continuous positive airway pressure on blood pressure in the sleep apnea-hypopnea syndrome. Am J Respir Crit Care Med 2001;163(2):344–8.

[11] Mayer J, Becker H, Brandenburg U, et al. Blood pressure and sleep apnea: results of long-term nasal continuous positive airway pressure therapy. Cardiology 1991;79(2):84–92.

[12] He J, Kryger MH, Zorick FJ, et al. Mortality and apnea index in obstructive sleep apnea. Experience in 385 male patients. Chest 1988;94(1):9–14.

[13] Berry RB, Parish JM, Hartse KM. The use of auto-titrating continuous positive airway pressure for treatment of adult obstructive sleep apnea. An American Academy of Sleep Medicine review. Sleep 2002;25(2):148–73.

[14] Meurice JC, Marc I, Series F. Efficacy of auto-CPAP in the treatment of obstructive sleep apnea/hypopnea syndrome. Am J Respir Crit Care Med 1996;153(2):794–8.

[15] d'Ortho MP, Grillier-Lanoir V, Levy P, et al. Constant vs. automatic continuous positive airway pressure therapy: home evaluation. Chest 2000; 118(4):1010–7.

[16] Sharma S, Wali S, Pouliot Z, et al. Treatment of obstructive sleep apnea with a self-titrating continuous positive airway pressure (CPAP) system. Sleep 1996;19(6):497–501.

[17] Stradling JR, Barbour C, Pitson DJ, et al. Automatic nasal continuous positive airway pressure titration in the laboratory: patient outcomes. Thorax 1997;52(1):72–5.

SLEEP
MEDICINE
CLINICS

Sleep Med Clin 1 (2006) 533–539

Positive Airway Pressure Adherence: Problems and Interventions

Mary W. Rose, PsyD, CBSM[a,b,*]

- Defining the problem
- Personality variables and compliance with continuous positive airway pressure
- Predictors of adherence problems
- Assessment of adherence
- Initiating intervention
- Intervention
- References

Defining the problem

Positive airway pressure therapy is the optimal treatment for the overwhelming majority of patients who have obstructive sleep apnea (OSA). The American Academy of Sleep Medicine Practice Parameters notes that CPAP is the first-line treatment for severe apnea [1]. Although oral appliances compare favorably with CPAP for treating mild-to-moderate OSA, oral appliances are not indicated for treating severe sleep apnea or sleep apnea accompanied by significant oxygen desaturations [2]. Despite the benefits of CPAP use, a significant proportion of patients are unable or unwilling to adhere to treatment. Before Smart Cards (devices that log a system's usage in detail) were developed, clinicians had only an overall hour-usage meter and patient self-reporting from which to estimate the duration of CPAP use. Reliance on self-reporting is precarious, at best. Previous research in the behavioral health arena (eg, diet and exercise program outcomes) consistently shows that self-reporting is exceedingly inaccurate. In one study, most patients reported regular use of CPAP, even though only 60% of that sample

reported using it 4.5 hours per night, or less in diaries [3]. These data suggest there are inconsistencies when the same subjects use different types of self-reporting. Likewise, Raucher and colleagues [4] found that patients who had poorer compliance consistently overestimated their total time of CPAP use.

Practitioners generally agree that not enough patients who could benefit from CPAP use it, and, among those who are receiving treatment, it generally is not used an optimal percentage of the time. The percentage of patients who are prescribed CPAP but who refuse treatment from onset is not well established. One study estimated such refusal as only about 5% [5]. Difficulty with the patient samples in the CPAP adherence research, nearly all of which is based on subjects who have at least initiated treatment, is that definitions of compliance vary, and there is no evidence that what is accepted is optimal or even adequate in treating a clinically significant proportion of the patients' apnea. Most definitions of adherence are defined as an average use of 4 or more hours per night for 70% of nights [6]; in other words, for one half of the total night

[a] Department of Medicine, Pulmonary and Critical Care Section, Baylor College of Medicine, 1 Baylor Plaza, Houston, TX 77030, USA
[b] Sleep Disorders & Research Center, Michael E. DeBakey Veterans Affairs Medical Center (111i), 2002 Holcombe Blvd., Houston, TX 77030, USA
* Correspondence. Sleep Center (111i), 2002 Holcombe Blvd., Bldg. 100, Rm 6C344, Houston, TX 77030.
E-mail address: mwrose@bcm.tmc.edu

doi:10.1016/j.jsmc.2006.10.005

70% of the time. Thus, at best, overall usage of CPAP is only about 35% of total sleep time. Studies generally do not report what times of night the unit is worn. Many patients treated by the author and colleagues have reported wearing the mask at the beginning of the night, and removing it at some time during the night, suggesting that these patients are untreated during REM sleep, when most of them have more disruptive and severe OSA events.

Accurate prescription of pressure, treatment of diurnal breathing problems that may affect mask usage (eg, nasal stuffiness), and a well-fitting mask, as well as education, are critical for compliance. Despite targeting all these factors, most centers see some rejection of initiating treatment, complete drop out, and a great majority of patients who use CPAP for, at best, one half of the night.

The innovation of the Smart Card has allowed clinicians to assess CPAP adherence objectively. Whether the knowledge of being monitored affects adherence is questionable. This technology does allow the clinician to identify patient management issues more quickly and accurately. Clinicians must remember that their ability to build rapport strengthens patients' accountability and investment into their own care; failure to build rapport may lead to a bitter and guarded patient who is less likely to be frank about health problems and less involved in his/her care. Thus, the interpretation of the Smart Card and the way these data are used and reviewed with the patient are important.

Long-term compliance estimates have ranged from less than 50% [6] to about 70% to 80% [7–11]. In one study compliance estimates were about 90% after 3 months [12]. In a sample of 50 patients, Ripberger and colleagues [13] and Krieger [14] found compliance of 90% after 5 years of treatment. Compliance of about 60% was found in adult males 65 and older [15].

Personality variables and compliance with continuous positive airway pressure

Edinger's [8] analysis showed the five predictors—sleepiness, overall sleep quality, body mass index, and elevations on the depression and hypochondriasis scales of the Minnesota Mutiphasic Personality Inventory (MMPI)—identify approximately 80% of eventual noncompliers and 97% of those who display compliance.

Edinger [8] found long-term use (defined as 6-month use) to be about 90% in 36 patients. Adherence was predicted by ANOVA using body mass index, sleepiness, subjective sleep quality, and elevations on MMPI depression and hypochondriasis scales. Thus, those who were compliant were heavier, less sleepy, had better sleep overall, and were less depressed and hypochondriacal before treatment. The finding regarding sleepiness and overall sleep quality is contrary to findings by others that patients who have unpleasant subjective symptoms are the ones who use CPAP, presumably because treatment has face validity for them. Indeed, most studies found sleepiness to be a critical predictor of CPAP adherence [16–18]. Edinger's group [8] speculated that the higher pretreatment scores on depression and hypochondriasis scales in noncompliant patients significantly influenced these patient's reports of greater sleepiness before treatment. Another study examining coping strategies found that those who had more active coping tendencies (eg, planful problem solving) were more likely to use CPAP. This active style of coping had greater predictive value than the respiratory distress index or daytime sleepiness [19]. These data suggest that personality styles may play a significant role in how an individual responds to treatment needs. Unlike mood disorder, personality is relatively fixed at an early age. Thus, if personality plays a major role in the individual's response to treatment, strategies for optimizing CPAP use based on personality barriers may be the next line of investigation in this area.

Chasens [20] found that patients who had high claustrophobia scores on a fear-avoidance scale had significantly more compliance problems with CPAP. One problematic assumption in this study was that fear avoidance is equated with claustrophobia. Alternatively, fear avoidance could be related less to claustrophobia and more to fear of acknowledging medical problems, especially if such acceptance requires use of a visually unappealing adaptive device, such as CPAP. Patients may be unable or unwilling to identify this source of their reluctance and default to blaming claustrophobia as a likely culprit for problems. These patients may be less likely to seek medical care, to take medications, or to receive routine testing. Patients who are self-conscious about their identity as independent or strong persons or who are young and single may be reluctant to accept CPAP. Emotionally, accepting treatment is acknowledgment of illness. Clinicians must compassionately examine these potential obstacles with patients.

Predictors of adherence problems

Predictors for and causes of CPAP noncompliance are discrete issues. The former involve largely measurable disease features, such as apnea-hypopnea index (AHI), body mass index, history of uvulopalatopharyngoplasty, oxygen desaturation level, and specific patient qualities, such as sex, age, and education. Causes for noncompliance are the reasons articulated by patients for being unable or unwilling to use CPAP. These causes usually include mask fit, feelings of suffocation from the pressure, nasal stuffiness, partner complaint about noise, cost, inconvenience for travel, or difficulty integrating the use of CPAP into one's identity.

As noted previously, the frequency and duration of CPAP use in the first month of treatment reliably predicted use in the third month [6]. Although the majority of patients interviewed claimed to use CPAP nightly, only 46% met the criteria for regular use, defined by at least 4 hours of CPAP administered, on 70% of the days monitored [6]. Another study found no predictors of compliance [21].

Research defining the predictors for noncompliance also is highly varied. Several studies found no difference in AHI [3,22]. CPAP level [3] and initial sleepiness [3,8] also have been poor predictors of compliance in some studies. Others found, to the contrary, that disease severity [23–25] and sleepiness [24] have a significant positive effect on compliance. Krieger's [14] study of 233 obstructive patients who had sleep apnea found disease severity to be significantly related to compliance. Those with lower education or with relatives already using CPAP seemed to have the greatest benefit [26].

Comparisons of those who dropped out early after initiating CPAP found compliers had a significantly higher AHI level [16,27], but noncompliers had significantly more severe oxygen desaturation levels. Aloia [28] found that patients who had greater baseline decrements in vigilance were more likely to use CPAP [28]. In a small sample, Kribbs [6] found that more frequent CPAP users tended to have more years of education.

Indeed, in the author's experience, the patient's indication of the likelihood of using CPAP does not seem to be related to how significantly its use affects the objective quality of sleep. All patients seen by the author and colleagues at the Veterans Administration Medical Center (VAMC) Sleep Center complete a survey the morning after their study that is used to evaluate candidacy for CPAP. Even excellent physical response to CPAP does not necessarily lead to compliance. Patients who generally have poor medical compliance, who do not understand the impact of apnea on their health, who refuse CPAP during titration, who report a history of claustrophobia, who are psychologically unsophisticated, or who are self conscious about using CPAP with a partner in the room are unlikely to be compliant.

Causes such as mouth breathing have been found to affect adherence negatively [29]. Becker [30] noted additional reasons included noise, pressure marks made by the mask, and intolerance to the high expiratory pressure. Patients have also complained of aerophagia. Some research has suggested that the type of airway pressure (C-flex or CPAP) [31] may affect compliance and provide a solution to some complaints related to pressure tolerance.

Assessment of adherence

After a sleep study, members of the author's group anticipate problems with compliance by querying patients about their experience with the system and possible problems they anticipate in using it. They ask

- **To what degree was your sleep improved?**
- **To what degree do you think CPAP will disturb your bed-partner?**
- **How likely are you to use CPAP?**

We have found the answers to these questions are a good predictor of CPAP use, and incorporate the patient's responses into their reports and our judgment as to whether the patient is a good candidate for CPAP.

When a patient returns to clinic, the physician provides him/her a copy of the report and reviews it with the patient. The physician highlights critical aspects of the study findings, explains that the patient stops breathing or significantly reduces breathing throughout the night and explain desaturations if the patient experiences them. We typically note to patients who have significant AHI and no desaturations that although their heart is strong and able to combat significant problems now, the apnea is putting an undue stress on them that CPAP may help alleviate. The author and her colleagues find it helpful to validate that many patients have difficulty adjusting to CPAP and that, if patients encounter problems, they should not give up but rather should work with the staff, who can help troubleshoot barriers. Validation is helpful in normalizing problems that arise, so the patient knows that coming for help is expected and that solutions are available.

The author's group also sees patients routinely every 6 months to evaluate usage, sleepiness, and recurrence of other possible symptoms, to check machine pressure, and to ensure that masks are in good working condition. Many of the patients at the VAMC Sleep Center were diagnosed elsewhere initially and report that no follow-up was ever scheduled for them at the clinic where they were seen initially. Often compliance barriers are solved by a mask change or an adjustment of the pressure delivery. The author's group checks patient machines routinely, because we have found more often than not that the machines are delivering pressure improperly. This finding may to be related to changes in barometric pressure in Houston, but it points out that clinics must be aware of the prevalence of re-set problems with CPAP in their areas.

Patients who report difficulty tolerating CPAP must be evaluated carefully to determine if the nature of the difficulty can be addressed through simple changes to the mask or head gear, by the addition of humidity, or by using bilevel positive airway pressure in lieu of CPAP. It is critical to identify patients who have primary claustrophobia, which may require additional treatment, probably cognitive behavioral therapy and/or psychopharmacologic treatment. We recommend against psychopharmacologic treatment of claustrophobia by the sleep clinician, because cognitive behavioral therapy is a first-line treatment and because claustrophobia is likely accompany other anxiety disorders and requires regular follow-up.

Initiating intervention

Chervin [26] compared interventions in the form of weekly telephone follow-up and problem-solving of CPAP problems with written educational materials. They found that both interventions improved CPAP compliance and were most salient when initiated during the first month of treatment.

Often the patient's medical problems are incorporated into the explanation regarding apnea, because many patients do not have a good understanding that major medical comorbidities are interactive and possibly synergistic. Commonly, patients experience medical conditions as completely independent of one another. Often the identification of an additional illness, such as apnea, is frustrating, and patient response may include reluctance to deal with additional treatments or illnesses. As do many sleep centers, the VAMC Sleep Center has a large population of patients who have diabetes, obesity, impotence, heart disease, and respiratory disease. In simple terms, the clinicians help patients understand how these diseases are tied with one another and that treating the apnea may lead to significant improvement in weight, diabetes management, metabolic control, and sexual and cardiac function.

Berry and Sanders [33] note several ways to improve adherence. These approaches include involvement of a spouse, extended-in-hospital stay, access to a positive airway pressure help line, unsolicited telephone follow-up, early intervention for side effects, objective monitoring, and regular clinic visits. The author and colleagues have found involvement of a spouse to be important, because

the spouse is the one who witnesses events, and for some patients a spouse's goading is the necessary catalyst for treatment. Spousal involvement also may remind the patient that his/her health is of paramount importance, above the inconveniences of the CPAP. Introducing CPAP to the inpatient allows monitored usage and assistance in troubleshooting. Identifying barriers that may prevent or delay a patient's getting CPAP and validating the treatment by its association with the medical reason for the inpatient admission are additional benefits. We refer nearly all patients to ear, nose, and throat specialists to ensure that there are no upper airway obstructions, allergy management, or other nasal issues that may prevent the patient from using CPAP. Many patients report removal of the mask during the night. The newly developed alarms are a useful strategy for identifying when patients remove their mask (information that can assist with troubleshooting why they do so) and for wakening the patient to replace the mask.

Intervention

Likar [32] provided a 2-hour group CPAP intervention for 73 male veterans who had OSA. Interventions were provided every 6 months and provided education, support, and equipment monitoring. Objective data were taken from patient machines; data for these patients suggested a significant increase of CPAP use, from 5.2 ± 0.6 to 6.3 ± 0.6 hours per night, after they had attended one or more CPAP clinics. These effects lasted for more than 18 months. Of patients receiving intervention, 29% increased nightly CPAP use by at least 2 hours; only 6% decreased use by 2 hours or more [32]. It is worth noting, however, that patient involvement in this clinic may suggest that they were already highly invested in treatment. In a small, randomized study, Aloia implemented cognitive behavioral therapy at 1-, 4-, and 12-week intervals after initiating treatment [24]. Patients in the treatment group received two individual sessions. Session one included cognitive tests, a review of symptoms and the advantages and disadvantages of treatment, and a review of sleep data. In the second session, compliance data were reviewed, and changes consequent to treatment, troubleshooting discomfort, and realistic goals and expectations were identified. Sleep data were evaluated without the subjects' awareness that it was being downloaded. Patients in the treatment group used CPAP significantly more (an additional 3.2 hours per night) than control subjects. This study showed that individualized structured intervention profoundly affects CPAP use for at least 12 weeks after baseline.

Many patients require CPAP desensitization to allow active troubleshooting of difficulty in adjusting to CPAP. The process of standard CPAP desensitization is relatively straightforward. Patients are interviewed to help identify the causes for their difficulty using CPAP. The first step in interviewing patients is to review the initial experience in the sleep laboratory. Unfortunately, technicians often do not prepare patients for the titration, and the first experience is one of confusion and discomfort. The titration process and rationale always should be explained carefully to the patient, both as a part of the initial consultation by the clinician and by the technician at the time of polysomnography. Such preparation has been shown to improve compliance significantly [34]. To avoid rapid discontinuation by the patient, it also should be explained that the airway has been "beaten up" by, perhaps, years of struggling to breathe, and that the patient may not feel benefits for up to 2 weeks. To ensure greater likelihood that the patient can imagine that the treatment will be useful in the long term, it also should be noted that the patient may experience an uncomfortable night even if benefits of CPAP are shown.

A number of approaches have been taken to improve adherence, including gradual titration during the day with problem solving throughout and weekly home instructions to desensitize gradually patients' discomfort or claustrophobic responses to CPAP. As noted previously, the first, indispensable step is to identify the reasons for problematic adherence. Desensitization is useful only in cases in which patients have difficulty adjusting to mask pressure or the aspects of the mask itself.

The author and colleagues have used the Maestro Clinical Remote (Respironics, Murrysville, Pennsylvania) for in-clinic desensitization. Although this approach typically takes several hours, it enables the clinician to identify the source of patient difficulty and to titrate the patient upward slowly. Sometimes patients are not able to clarify the sensation that is causing difficulty unless they are experiencing CPAP. Patients tend to be more articulate about difficulty in exhaling (in lieu of simply describing the sensation of "suffocating" while being titrated); patients who describe difficulty in exhaling may be good candidates for bilevel positive airway pressure. Having the patient in the laboratory also detaches the patient from the home environment in which the patient has established psychophysiologic arousal cues and tests the patient's belief that he/she cannot sleep with the machine. A patient may see that he/she is able to fall asleep successfully. Often, validating that this task is accomplishable but challenging is important for successful titration.

Inevitably there will be patients who have histories of abuse or chronic nightmares that may significantly complicate desensitization. Although occasionally there are unexpected reasons for difficulty in using CPAP, the author and colleague have found these issues to be just below the surface and readily open for discussion. One of their patients was resistant to CPAP because her husband, who had an extremely complicated medical history, had started CPAP therapy shortly before his death. When the patient was diagnosed, she felt that accepting treatment was a path to her own death and that CPAP must be ineffective because it did not save her husband. Dispelling misunderstandings about the function of CPAP and acknowledging its limitations in combination with grief counseling were important in enabling this patient to initiate her treatment. Another patient, an elderly man who lived alone, was unable to use CPAP because his primary care physician, in attempt to pre-empt adherence problems, told him that he would die if he did not treat his apnea. Unfortunately this statement caused serious anxiety, with the consequence that the patient developed insomnia and anxiety with hypnic jerks that he believed were consequent to apneic events that were leading to his ultimate demise. For this patient, reassurance that he would not die from apnea while falling asleep in his lounger and decatastrophizing his condition helped diminish his anxiety surrounding sleep, his insomnia, and his difficulty in getting to sleep with his unit. It is particularly important to recall that OSA has a high comorbidity with depression. Because apneics are just as likely as any other patient to have poor sleep hygiene, circadian problems, sleep restriction, and occasional to chronic insomnia, addressing these issues is often of critical importance in establishing CPAP compliance successfully. In fact, with the second patient, loneliness and need for a pet became a central focus of therapy. Many months after he was treated, he called to inform the author and colleagues that he was using his CPAP vigilantly and had obtained a new cat.

Education may affect CPAP compliance significantly. Like many centers, the VAMC Sleep Center runs a brief video in the waiting room that follows a patient from the time of considering assessment through evaluation and treatment. This video prepares patients for the interview and provides a recognizable scenario with which they often can identify. One study has found such videos to have a significant positive effect on compliance [35].

It is important to explain that many patients experience some anxiety in adjusting to CPAP.

For patients who are defensive about their need for CPAP, the author and colleagues typically normalize treatment by speaking in broad terms about the symptom relief reported by other patients. Often a quick review of patient comorbidities can help the patient focus on the ways in which CPAP may be of direct benefit to the patent's other health concerns. Understanding that the airway often is edematous and that it may take a few weeks to experience perceived improved quality of sleep prepares patients and may avoid premature termination of treatment when immediate results are not experienced.

Assumptions related to the causes of compliance problems and how compliance is defined leave much to be desired. As in many aspects of health care, the complexities that behavior and emotion bring to the equation are often neglected. For centers that have a behavioral sleep specialist, the initial session is spent building rapport and identifying likely psychologic and physical contributors to the patient's difficulty with adherence. A careful psychologic evaluation to understand the role of comorbid mood disorders and self-image issues is of critical importance. Patients who are anxious or depressed may have a decreased ability to manage a medical challenge. Anxiety tends to lead to agitation, and depression often leads to apathy. As with good psychotherapy, the factors that enable effective treatment of CPAP adherence problems are empathy and rapport.

References

[1] Thorpy M, Einstein A, Derderian S, et al. Practice parameters for the treatment of snoring and obstructive sleep-apnea with oral appliances. Sleep 1995;18(6):511–3.

[2] Kushida CA, Littner MR, Morgenthaler T, et al. Practice parameters for the indications for polysomnography and related procedures: an update for 2005. Sleep 2005;28(4):499–521.

[3] Alarcon A, Leon C, Maimo A, et al. [Compliance with nasal continuous positive airway pressure (CPAP) treatment in sleep apnea-hypopnea syndrome]. Arch Bronconeumol 1995;31(2):56–61. [in Spanish].

[4] Rauscher H, Formanek D, Popp W, et al. Self-reported vs measured compliance with nasal CPAP for obstructive sleep apnea. Chest 1993;103(6): 1675–80.

[5] McArdle N, Devereux G, Heidarnejad H, et al. Long-term use of CPAP therapy for sleep apnea/hypopnea syndrome. Am J Respir Crit Care Med 1999;159(4 Pt 1):1108–14.

[6] Kribbs NB, Pack AI, Kline LR, et al. Objective measurement of patterns of nasal CPAP use by patients with obstructive sleep apnea. Am Rev Respir Dis 1993;147(4):887–95.

[7] Pepin JL, Krieger J, Rodenstein D, et al. Effective compliance during the first 3 months of continuous positive airway pressure. A European prospective study of 121 patients. Am J Respir Crit Care Med 1999;160(4):1124–9.

[8] Edinger JD, Carwile S, Miller P, et al. Psychological status, syndromatic measures, and compliance with nasal CPAP therapy for sleep apnea. Percept Mot Skills 1994;78(3 Pt 2): 1116–8.

[9] Hohenhaus-Beer A, Gleixner M, Fichter J. [Long-term follow-up of CPAP therapy in patients with obstructive sleep apnea]. Wien Med Wochenschr 1995;145(17–18):512–4 [in German].

[10] Marquez-Baez C, Paniagua-Soto J, Castilla-Garrido JM. [Treatment of sleep apnea syndrome with CPAP: compliance with treatment, its efficacy and secondary effects]. Rev Neurol 1998;26(151):375–80 [in Spanish].

[11] Parish JM, Lyng PJ, Wisbey J. Compliance with CPAP in elderly patients with OSA. Sleep Med 2000;1(3):209–14.

[12] Krieger J, Kurtz D. Objective measurement of compliance with nasal CPAP treatment for obstructive sleep apnoea syndrome. Eur Respir J 1988;1(5):436–8.

[13] Ripberger R, Pirsig W. [Nasal positive pressure ventilation (nCPAP) in therapy of obstructive sleep apnea: acceptance by 50 patients]. Laryngorhinootologie 1994;73(11):581–5 [in German].

[14] Krieger J. Long-term compliance with nasal continuous positive airway pressure (CPAP) in obstructive sleep apnea patients and nonapneic snorers. Sleep 1992;15(6 Suppl):S42–6.

[15] Russo-Magno P, O'Brien A, Panciera T, et al. Compliance with CPAP therapy in older men with obstructive sleep apnea. J Am Geriatr Soc 2001;49(9):1205–11.

[16] Rauscher H, Popp W, Wanke T, et al. Acceptance of CPAP therapy for sleep apnea. Chest 1991; 100(4):1019–23.

[17] Rolfe I, Olson LG, Saunders NA. Long-term acceptance of continuous positive airway pressure in obstructive sleep apnea. Am Rev Respir Dis 1991;144(5):1130–3.

[18] Sanders MH, Gruendl CA, Rogers RM. Patient compliance with nasal CPAP therapy for sleep apnea. Chest 1986;90(3):330–3.

[19] Stepnowsky CJ Jr, Bardwell WA, Moore PJ, et al. Psychologic correlates of compliance with continuous positive airway pressure. Sleep 2002; 25(7):758–62.

[20] Chasens ER, Pack AI, Maislin G, et al. Claustrophobia and adherence to CPAP treatment. West J Nurs Res 2005;27(3):307–21.

[21] Reeves-Hoche MK, Meck R, Zwillich CW. Nasal CPAP: an objective evaluation of patient compliance. Am J Respir Crit Care Med 1994;149(1): 149–54.

[22] Engleman HM, Martin SE, Douglas NJ. Compliance with CPAP therapy in patients with the sleep apnoea/hypopnoea syndrome. Thorax 1994; 49(3):263–6.

[23] Meurice JC, Dore P, Paquereau J, et al. Predictive factors of long-term compliance with nasal continuous positive airway pressure treatment in sleep apnea syndrome. Chest 1994;105(2):429–33.

[24] Dong X, He Q, Han F, et al. The compliance with nasal continuous positive airway pressure in patients with sleep apnea syndrome. Zhonghua Jie He He Hu Xi Za Zhi 2002;25(7):399–402.

[25] Hui DS, Choy DK, Li TS, et al. Determinants of continuous positive airway pressure compliance in a group of Chinese patients with obstructive sleep apnea. Chest 2001;120(1):170–6.

[26] Chervin RD, Theut S, Bassetti C, et al. Compliance with nasal CPAP can be improved by simple interventions. Sleep 1997;20(4):284–9.

[27] Janson C, Noges E, Svedberg-Randt S, et al. What characterizes patients who are unable to tolerate continuous positive airway pressure (CPAP) treatment? Respir Med 2000;94(2):145–9.

[28] Aloia MS, Ilniczky N, Di DP, et al. Neuropsychological changes and treatment compliance in older adults with sleep apnea. J Psychosom Res 2003;54(1):71–6.

[29] Bachour A, Maasilta P. Mouth breathing compromises adherence to nasal continuous positive airway pressure therapy. Chest 2004;126(4):1248–54.

[30] Becker H, Fett I, Nees E, et al. [Treatment of primary and secondary therapy failure in patients with sleep apnea treated with nasal CPAP]. Pneumologie 1991;45(Suppl 1):301–5 [in German].

[31] Aloia MS, Stanchina M, Arnedt JT, et al. Treatment adherence and outcomes in flexible vs standard continuous positive airway pressure therapy. Chest 2005;127(6):2085–93.

[32] Likar LL, Panciera TM, Erickson AD, et al. Group education sessions and compliance with nasal CPAP therapy. Chest 1997;111(5):1273–7.

[33] Berry RB, Sanders MH. Positive airway pressure treatment for sleep apnea. In: Carney PR, Berry RB, Geyer JD, editors. Clinical sleep disorders. Philadelphia: Lippincott Williams & Williams; 2005. p. 290–310.

[34] Means MK, Edinger JD, Husain AM. CPAP compliance in sleep apnea patients with and without laboratory CPAP titration. Sleep Breath 2004;8(1):7–14.

[35] Jean WH, Boethel C, Phillips B, et al. CPAP compliance: video education may help! Sleep Med 2005;6(2):171–4.

ELSEVIER
SAUNDERS

SLEEP
MEDICINE
CLINICS

Sleep Med Clin 1 (2006) 541–548

Perioperative Management of Obstructive Sleep Apnea

Charlie K. Lan, DO, DABSM[a,b,*], Mary W. Rose, PsyD, CBSM[a]

- Effects of sedatives, anesthetics, and analgesic agents on the respiratory system
- Other factors contributing to perioperative risk
- Diagnosing and evaluating sleep apnea in the preoperative period
- Clinical considerations in patients who have obstructive sleep apnea

- *Preoperative considerations*
- *Intraoperative considerations*
- *Postoperative considerations*
- Management
- *Preoperative management*
- *Intraoperative management*
- *Postoperative management*
- References

Obstructive sleep apnea syndrome (OSA) is a common disorder. The estimated prevalence of sleep-disordered breathing is about 2% for women and 4% for men between the ages of 30 and 60 years [1,2]. Furthermore, OSA is underdiagnosed in an estimated 80% of patients [3]. Most attention on OSA in recent years has been focused on the significantly increased risk of hypertension, cardiac arrhythmia [4–6], pulmonary hypertension [7,8], right heart failure [4,7,9], myocardial infarction [4,10,11], and stroke [12–17].

Few data exist in the literature examining the effects of OSA on perioperative complications and management. In addition, in one survey study of anesthesiologists, 72% reported no departmental policy on management of patients who have OSA [2]. This lack is quite astonishing given the significant morbidity and mortality associated with the airway compromise caused by anesthesia and perioperative medications.

As OSA becomes a better-recognized disease, the relationship between OSA and complications from anesthesia and postoperative analgesia has gained wider attention [18,19]. The role of OSA as a risk factor for anesthetic morbidity and mortality is considerable [18,20–25]. The perioperative risks associated with OSA can be primary or secondary. The primary perioperative risk factors associated with OSA include collapsed upper airway, hypoxemia, associated pathophysiologic change, and difficult airway control. Secondary causes include underlying obesity or abnormal upper airway anatomy [25,26]. The secondary risks involve associated comorbidities such as cardiovascular diseases. All vulnerabilities to apnea are enhanced during the period of sedation by either anesthesia or analgesia use [21,23–26].

To date, there are some data on perioperative complications and management of patients who have OSA related to surgical correction of the upper airway [27–31]. Less is known about perioperative complications and management of patients who have OSA undergoing non–upper airway surgery [32,33], but increasing evidence supports a link

[a] Department of Medicine, Pulmonary and Critical Care Section, Baylor College of Medicine, 1 Baylor Plaza, Houston, TX 77030, USA
[b] Sleep Disorders & Research Center, Michael E. DeBakey Veterans Affairs Medical Center (111i), 2002 Holcombe Blvd., Houston, TX 77030, USA
* Corresponding author. Baylor College of Medicine MED VAMC, Building 100 (111i), Houston, TX 77030, USA
E-mail address: clan@bcm.tmc.edu (C.K. Lan).

1556-407X/06/$ – see front matter © 2006 Elsevier Inc. All rights reserved.
sleep.theclinics.com

doi:10.1016/j.jsmc.2006.11.004

between postoperative complications in patients who have OSA who received anesthesia and analgesia for non–upper airway surgery. Increased recognition of these potential complications has slowly modified the way physicians manage patients who have OSA during peri- and postoperative care. A recent survey of Canadian anesthesiologists demonstrated a high frequency of caring for patients with OSA, either diagnosed or undiagnosed [2]. Most of the anesthesiologists surveyed had personally experienced complications associated with OSA. Unfortunately, most centers do not have departmental policies in guiding the management of patients who have OSA [2], even though a majority of anesthesiologists surveyed believed that such guidelines would assist them in providing care to patients who have OSA [2].

Effects of sedatives, anesthetics, and analgesic agents on the respiratory system

OSA is a heterogeneous disease associated with sleep fragmentation and often hypoxemia. In many patients who have OSA, upper airway size is diminished by enlarged tonsils, a low or narrow arched soft palate, or a thick tongue. Retrognathia and micrognathia may further compromise the airway and contribute to narrowing of the airway during sleep. In patients who have OSA, lung volume decreases and airway resistance increases during sleep, independent of the degree of obesity [34]. The perioperative risks associated with OSA may result from a number of different factors including a collapsed upper airway, hypoxemia, associated pathophysiologic changes, difficult airway control secondary to underlying obesity or abnormal upper airway anatomy, or associated comorbidities such as cardiovascular disease. These risks increase preoperatively because of the direct and indirect effects of sedatives, analgesics, and anesthetic agents on the upper airway, respiratory system, and central nervous system. Furthermore, patients who have OSA seem to be much more sensitive to the effects of sedation and analgesia [35].

The agents used perioperatively for sedation and analgesia reduce functional residual capacity, predispose to atelectasis [36,37], increase upper airway collapsibility, and reduce ventilatory response to hypoxemia and hypercapnia [38,39]. These responses can worsen the severity of underlying OSA. Sedation and analgesics can further induce sleep apnea in patients who otherwise do not have clinically significant OSA, decrease arousal and ventilatory response to respiratory events, and worsen hypoxemia. Sedative-, anesthetic-, and analgesic-related disturbances in patients who have

OSA may persist into the postoperative period. The persistent effects of these medications may warrant the close monitoring of patients who have OSA for several days postoperatively.

Cardiovascular complications related to hypoxemia and increased risk of pneumonia associated with atelectasis are significantly increased peri- and postoperatively. Arousal from sleep is an important defense mechanism that occurs during natural sleep to overcome the upper airway collapse in patients who have OSA. This mechanism is absent or blunted in patients who are under the influence of sedatives, anesthetics, and analgesic agents, potentially leading to life-threatening consequences.

Table 1 lists the general and local effects of anesthetics, sedatives, and analgesic agents on the human respiratory system. The agents depress consciousness, reduce arousal response, decrease skeletal muscle tone [40,41], diminish neural input to upper airway tone [41], and inhibit respiration. Upper airway patency depends on multiple factors, including anatomic characteristics, tonic and phasic upper airway muscle activity, and thoracic volume. Immediately before contraction of diaphragm, phasic activity and contraction of the pharyngeal dilator muscles increases upper airway tone and thus prevents collapse of the upper airway [38,42]. Phasic activity of the pharyngeal muscle is diminished significantly by the administration of anesthetic and analgesic drugs [43].

***Table 1:* Effects of sedative, anesthetic, and analgesics on the respiratory system**

General effect	Local effects
CNS depression	Depressed consciousness Reduced arousal responses Decreased skeletal muscle tone Decreased upper airway tone Reduced neural input to upper airway muscle
Respiratory depression Ventilatory depression	Decreased functional residue capacity Diminished ventilatory response to hypoxemia and hypercapnia
Respiratory workload depression	Reduced response to elastic and resistive workload

Data from: Refs. [36–38,40,42,64–66].

Other factors contributing to perioperative risk

Other factors besides the effects of anesthetics, sedatives, and analgesic agents may contribute to increased perioperative risk. Most patients experience sleep deprivation perioperatively because of anticipation of the surgery, anxiety, and conditions related to the surgery, pain, and medications. Sleep deprivation exacerbates OSA and thus increases the peri- and postoperative complications associated with OSA.

Immediately after surgery, total sleep time, slow-wave sleep, and rapid eye movement (REM) sleep significantly diminish because of pain, postoperative analgesic use, and hormonal and metabolic changes [44–46]. Recovery of these disturbances in sleep architecture may take as long as a week [46]. Consequent to sleep deprivation, slow-wave and REM sleep rebound immediately postoperatively. Sleep apneic events tend to be more frequent and severe during this period of recovery and can cause more significant hypoxemia. This hypoxemia has been shown to be associated with increased cardiovascular events, poor wound healing, mental confusion, and surgical delirium [47].

Diagnosing and evaluating sleep apnea in the preoperative period

Preoperative evaluation of any patient should include an assessment of the likelihood of OSA. In previously diagnosed patients, a copy of the diagnostic and therapeutic sleep studies should be reviewed thoroughly. Information such as the apnea-hypopnea index, oxygen saturation nadir, associated arrhythmias, sleep architecture, effect of body position [48], treatment modality (continuous positive airway pressure [CPAP], bilevel positive airway pressure, an oral appliance, or upper airway surgery), type of interface (nasal or full-face mask), pressure requirement, and need for supplemental oxygen should be reviewed thoroughly to understand the nature and severity of the patient's OSA. This information provides an important guide for peri- and postoperative management. A patient who has previously undergone upper airway surgery for OSA should be evaluated for current symptoms, because there is a significant rate of postsurgical relapse [49]. Continued presence or recurrence of OSA symptoms after any treatment should be assessed, especially if there is a significant change in patient's body weight or medications. If there are continued OSA symptoms in patients who have been treated, a repeat therapeutic or titration sleep study should be done before the surgery.

Often the anesthesiologist sees the patient only during the preoperative evaluation. It is therefore important for anesthesiologist to inquire about OSA and identify patients who might have OSA to address the proper peri- and postoperative management to prevent the complication associated with OSA [50]. Because often the time the anesthesiologist spends with a patient for preoperative evaluation is brief, it is crucial to have a concise but systemic way of identifying possible OSA. A questionnaire may prove a useful and efficient way to ensure consistency in identifying preoperatively patients who have OSA. Table 2 provides a list of questions that may be used during a brief patient encounter to identify and assess quickly patients who may have symptoms of OSA. Some are commonly used apnea-screening questions; some were included in the American Academy of Sleep Medicine recommendations for OSA screening; and some the authors commonly use in their screening instruments. The absence of positive responses to the questions in Table 2 or of the characteristics in Box 1 does not eliminate the possibility of OSA.

Box 1 lists the characteristics associated with a high risk of OSA. This list can be used during a brief encounter to identify at-risk patients quickly. If time allows, or if the patient is undergoing an elective surgery, the surgery should be postponed until a proper sleep evaluation and study has been done and sleep apnea treated. For urgent surgery, the patient should be assumed to have OSA.

Clinical considerations in patients who have obstructive sleep apnea

Preoperative considerations

Intuitively, control of comorbid conditions before anesthesia reduces complications resulting from anesthesia and surgery. Thus, adequate treatment of OSA before anesthesia may reduce complications. To the authors' knowledge, however, there are no published studies evaluating the effect of preoperative intervention that may improve adherence to apnea treatment (eg, weight loss, mandibular advancement, use of CPAP) on postoperative morbidity. In the nonanesthesia setting, CPAP has been shown to improve sympathetic nerve activity [51,52]. Diurnal blood pressure also has been shown to improve significantly with CPAP treatment of patients who have OSA [51,53,54]. The effect of CPAP therapy on hypertension may be limited to hypertensive patients who have excessive sleepiness, however [55].

Numerous red flags suggest the need for preoperative evaluation for apnea. Ideally, before surgery, care providers should feel confident that patients who have apnea have been diagnosed and properly

Table 2: Brief questionnaire for identifying risk of obstructive sleep apnea

Do you snore nightly?	Y	N
Do you wake up middle of night with shortness of breath, choking, or gasping for air?	Y	N
Do others tell you that you stop breathing while you sleep?	Y	N
Do you wake up in the morning feeling unrefreshed?	Y	N
Do you often wake up in the morning with a headache?	Y	N
Do you have difficulty breathing through your nose?	Y	N
Do you fall asleep easily during the day?	Y	N

titrated before the surgery. Unfortunately, many patients are undiagnosed or inadequately treated. Additionally, many patients have had airway surgery to treat apnea that may not have been successful or may even have resulted in structural changes that have compromised the airway. In addition to the standard review of medical records, all patients

Box 1: Characteristics highly associated with obstructive sleep apnea

Male sex
Body mass index > 25 kg/m^2
Physical characteristics
High mellampati airway stage
Short and large neck circumference
>17 inches in men
>16 inches in women
Narrow oropharynx (large tonsils, redundant pharyngeal arches)
Hypertrophy of nasal turbinate
Retrognathia
Macroglossia
Enlarged tonsils
Habitual snoring and gasping reported by bed partner
Witnessed apnea
Daytime sleepiness
Hypertension

Data from: Refs. [41,54–59,67–71].

should be interviewed for possible apnea and receive and airway evaluation. If possible, the presence of a bed partner during the preoperative evaluation can be extremely helpful, because patients often are unaware of symptoms that may be noted by their partner.

The guidelines developed by the American Society of Anesthesiologists task force recommend that patients who possess two of the following characteristics should be assumed to have moderate OSA:

1. Clinical signs and symptoms suggestive of OSA
2. History of apparent airway obstruction
3. Somnolence

Further, the American Society of Anesthesiologists notes that severe manifestations of any of these symptoms should be treated as though severe apnea is present. The task force had provided a rough screening tool for sleep apnea to assist providers in making judgments about the treatment of potential OSA [56].

Some health benefits of CPAP do not become apparent until several months of use. For example, Shivalkar [57] found that patients who have OSA showed significant evidence of improved hemodynamics and left and right ventricular morphology and function after 6 months of CPAP use. Several other parameters show rapid response to CPAP, however. Glucose regulation is profoundly affected by apnea. Blood glucose levels are elevated in nondiabetic patients treated with CPAP for 1 night [58]. Optimal preoperative benefit of CPAP may require 4 to 6 weeks of treatment for edema in the airway to subside [59]. Improvement of sympathetic activity and blood pressure within 24 hours is promising, because most generally noncompliant patients may be able to adhere to CPAP use more rigorously if asked to focus on use for at least the few days before surgery. If the role of evaluating and implementing a plan falls upon the anesthesiologist, the ability of CPAP to improve symptoms within 24 hours of usage becomes more important, because the patient may be seen for this appointment only 24 hours before surgery.

Many of the authors' patients have noted in interview that it was a physician who witnessed their apnea, hearing or seeing them in their room during a surgical admission. Prescreening is crucial to prepare presurgically and to optimize recovery after surgery. Preoperative screening should be viewed as a necessary step to avoid complications perioperatively and during recovery and as an opportunity to identify a previously undiagnosed medical problem that if treated would likely lead to improvement in overall outcome from any surgery and in overall quality of life.

For patients who have been diagnosed as having apnea, reviewing their adherence to CPAP provides an opportunity to remind patients that their active involvement in care and health behavior is crucial to their recovery.

Thus, preoperatively, patient should be assessed for the presence OSA and the adequacy of OSA therapy. Optimization of OSA treatment may reduce perioperative complications.

Intraoperative considerations

The intraoperative care and monitoring of the patient who has OSA should follow guidelines similar to those for obese and airway-compromised patients. Although patients under general anesthesia are ventilated, both intubation and extubation pose especially difficult perioperative problems. In patients who have severe OSA or significant airway compromise, preoperative intubation and postoperative extubation during wake is highly recommended. This technique will help avoid a panic and prolonged attempt to access an airway that has become more difficult to access consequent to a preintubation sedation.

Patients often are heavily sedated, and the postoperative regimen often includes narcotics, sedatives, and hypnotics. Patients who have not been using CPAP regularly or for long enough may still have airway edema.

Further, the supine position during perioperative period may worsen upper airway obstruction. After evaluation of 80 upright and supine cephalograms, Pae [60] observed that pharyngeal length in the supine position compared with the upright position seemed to be more important than the measurement of the most constricted area of the pharynx alone in the diagnosis and treatment of OSA. In morbidly obese subjects, expiratory flow is limited when the subject is in the supine position [61]. Patients continue to have impaired respiratory response to hypoxemia following surgery, and impairment of ventilatory and cardiovascular responses to hypoxia is much greater in patients compromised by cardiopulmonary diseases.

Postoperative considerations

Patients who have apnea should be given special attention during extubation, because as this process presents multiple risks for airway-compromised patients. Because anesthesia, antiemetics, and postoperative pain medications dramatically affect sleep architecture, they should be used only as needed. As noted previously, these medications often decrease pharyngeal tone and consequently arousal from hypoxia and hypercapnia. Shorter-acting hypnotics may thus be preferred.

Immediately after surgery, the use of CPAP may be indicated. Because of increased REM rebound, and continued sedation, patients are even more vulnerable to obstruction. Special attention should be paid to the possibility of vomiting and aspiration of stomach content during CPAP use. Patients who use CPAP only rarely or who tend to travel without it are unlikely to bring the device to the hospital for perioperative use. Medical staff should remind patients to bring their machine and have a family member bring it in if the patient does not do so.

Management

Preoperative management

Preoperative screening should include a careful interview of CPAP use. Patients are notoriously inaccurate in their reports of CPAP usage. If the physician emphases CPAP use as a critical step to maximize preoperative status, however, patients are likely to use their CPAP device more diligently. This situation is an opportunistic time to re-evaluate compliance and perhaps have the patient return to the sleep clinician or to be referred to a behavioral sleep expert to address adherence obstacles. Many patients have been lost to follow-up and are unaware that significant changes in weight, aging, and development of nasal allergies can contribute to a need for a change in CPAP pressure. The authors have often worked with patients who stopped using CPAP because they thought it had cured their apnea. Physicians may wish to focus on one or two simple take-home messages to improve patients' use of CPAP.

Change is a grueling task for most people, and the physician must be cautious in choosing where they place their emphasis for patient adherence. Realistically, issues of adherence that are not perceived by the patient as having an obvious benefit or that require extended or unpleasant activities will meet with greater noncompliance. Likewise, patients are more likely to focus on medical needs that their care providers have significantly and frequently emphasized.

Reduction in anesthetic dose may be helpful in patients who have OSA. Pawlik [62] found that clonidine given the night before and 2 hours before surgery augmented the efficacy of a smaller dose of surgical anesthetic. Mean arterial blood pressures were significantly lower during induction, operation, and emergence from anesthesia. In the group receiving clonidine, propofol doses required befor and during surgery were significantly reduced compared with the placebo group. Piritramide consumption and analgesia scores also were significantly reduced [62].

Because of the sedating property of clonidine can worsen OSA, but it is efficacious in reducing the need for intraoperative anesthetics, the preoperative strategy of prescribing CPAP the night before surgery in patients suspected of having OSA and who will be administered clonidine may be warranted. Among the benefits of reducing the amount of required anesthetic is a significant improvement of sleep architecture during the period of postoperative recovery.

Intraoperative management

Surgery involving conscious sedation poses significant vulnerability for airway closure. The practice guidelines for perioperative management of patients who have OSA outline risk factors for respiratory depression in these patients: systemic and neuraxial administration of opioids, administration of sedatives, the severity of the patient's apnea, and the invasiveness and site of the surgery [54]. This task force makes a number of recommendations regarding perioperative anesthesia management of the patient who has OSA. The guidelines are highly recommended reading for anyone desiring general guidelines on patient management.

Postoperative management

Patients who have OSA often have extremely sensitive airways. Any postoperative medication that depresses central nervous system activity could lead to significant worsening of symptoms. The practice guidelines for perioperative management of patients who have OSA suggest a full reversal of neuromuscular block and an awake state before extubation [63]. Preferably, the patient should be extubated in a nonsupine position. The guidelines further recommend using regional anesthetics rather than systemic opioids, with preference given to nonsteroidal anti-inflammatory agents.

Patient response to measures designed to minimize complications from OSA should be well documented for future surgeries and to emphasize that OSA is a condition requiring nightly attention, not just temporary attention in response to a surgical need.

In summary, OSA is a prevalent disease, and many patients who undergo surgery suffer from OSA. It's presence increases the risk of perioperative complications. Thus, preoperative evaluation should include assessment for the presence of OSA and the adequacy of the patient's current treatment. Optimization of OSA therapy preoperatively may reduce perioperative complications related to OSA. Special attention to the use of sedatives and analgesics is important in these patients. Postoperatively, prolonged monitoring and the use of CPAP may be indicated. Ultimately, a well-developed protocol for perioperative evaluation and management of patients who have OSA may reduce perioperative complications.

References

[1] Young T, Palta M, Dempsey J, et al. The occurrence of sleep-disordered breathing among middle-aged adults. N Engl J Med 1993;328(17): 1230–5.

[2] Turner K, VanDenkerkhof E, Lam M, et al. Perioperative care of patients with obstructive sleep apnea—a survey of Canadian anesthesiologists. Can J Anaesth 2006;53(3):299–304.

[3] Young T, Evans L, Finn L, et al. Estimation of the clinically diagnosed proportion of sleep apnea syndrome in middle-aged men and women. Sleep 1997;20(9):705–6.

[4] Coccagna G, Pollini A, Provini F. Cardiovascular disorders and obstructive sleep apnea syndrome. Clin Exp Hypertens 2006;28(3–4):217–24.

[5] Grimm W, Becker HF. Obesity, sleep apnea syndrome, and rhythmogenic risk. Herz 2006;31(3): 213–8.

[6] Mehra R, Benjamin EJ, Shahar E, et al. Association of nocturnal arrhythmias with sleep-disordered breathing—the Sleep Heart Health Study. Am J Respir Crit Care Med 2006;173(8):910–6.

[7] Rasche K, Orth M, Duchna HW. Sequels of lung diseases on cardiac function. Med Klin 2006;101: 44–6.

[8] Kessler R, Chaouat A, Weitzenblum E, et al. Pulmonary hypertension in the obstructive sleep apnoea syndrome: prevalence, causes and therapeutic consequences. Eur Respir J 1996;9(4): 787–94.

[9] Bradley TD, Rutherford R, Grossman RF, et al. Role of daytime hypoxemia in the pathogenesis of right heart-failure in the obstructive sleep-apnea syndrome. Am Rev Respir Dis 1985;131(6): 835–9.

[10] Sanner B, Sturm A, Konermann M. Coronary heart disease in patients with obstructive sleep apnoea. Dtsch Med Wochenschr 1996;121(30): 931–5.

[11] Shepard JW. Symposium on sleep disorders. 4. Cardiopulmonary consequences of obstructive sleep-apnea. Mayo Clin Proc 1990;65(9): 1250–9.

[12] Ferini-Strambi L, Fantini ML. Cerebrovascular diseases and sleep-disordered breathing. Clin Exp Hypertens 2006;28(3–4):225–31.

[13] Brown DL. Sleep disorders and stroke. Semin Neurol 2006;26(1):117–22.

[14] Elwood P, Hack M, Pickering J, et al. Sleep disturbance, stroke, and heart disease events: evidence from the Caerphilly cohort. J Epidemiol Community Health 2006;60(1):69–73.

[15] Yaggi HK, Concato J, Kernan WN, et al. Obstructive sleep apnea as a risk factor for stroke and death. N Engl J Med 2005;353(19):2034–41.

[16] Yang HG, You G, Zhu S. [The relationship between sleep related breathing disorders and stroke]. Zhonghua Jie He He Hu Xi Za Zhi 1999;22(6):341–3 [in Chinese].

[17] Munoz R. Severe sleep apnea and risk for ischemic stroke in the elderly. Stroke 2006;37(9): 2317–21.

[18] Hartmann B, Junger A, Klasen J. Anesthesia and sleep apnea syndrome. Anaesthesist 2005; 54(7):684.

[19] Hiremath AS, Hillman DR, James AL, et al. Relationship between difficult tracheal intubation and obstructive sleep apnoea. Br J Anaesth 1998;80(5):606–11.

[20] Moos DD, Cuddeford JD. Implications of obstructive sleep apnea syndrome for the perianesthesi nurse. J Perianesth Nurs 2006;21(2):103–15.

[21] Deutzer J. Potential complications of obstructive sleep apnea in patients undergoing gastric bypass surgery. Crit Care Nurs Q 2005;28(3):293–9.

[22] Jarrell L. Perioperative diagnosis and postoperative management of adult patients with obstructive sleep apnea syndrome: a review of the literature. J Perianesth Nurs 1999;14(4): 193–200.

[23] Esclamado RM, Glenn MG, McCulloch TM, et al. Perioperative complications and risk factors in the surgical treatment of obstructive sleep apnea syndrome. Laryngoscope 1989;99(11):1125–9.

[24] Benumof JL. Obstructive sleep apnea in the adult obese patient: implications for airway management. Anesthesiol Clin North America 2002; 20(4):789–811.

[25] Moos DD, Prasch M, Cantral DE, et al. Are patients with obstructive sleep apnea syndrome appropriate candidates for the ambulatory surgical center? AANA J 2005;73(3):197–205.

[26] Kim JA, Lee JJ, Jung HH. Predictive factors of immediate postoperative complications after uvulopalatopharyngoplasty. Laryngoscope 2005; 115(10):1837–40.

[27] Statham MM. Adenotonsillectomy for obstructive sleep apnea syndrome in young children: prevalence of pulmonary complications. Arch Otolaryngol Head Neck Surg 2006;132(5):476–80.

[28] Regli A, von Ungern-Sternberg BS, Strobel WM, et al. The impact of postoperative nasal packing on sleep-disordered breathing and nocturnal oxygen saturation in patients with obstructive sleep apnea syndrome. Anesth Analg 2006;102(2): 615–20.

[29] Pavone M, Paglietti MG, Petrone A, et al. Adenotonsillectomy for obstructive sleep apnea in children with Prader-Willi syndrome. Pediatr Pulmonol 2006;41(1):74–9.

[30] Li RH, Zeng Y, Wang YJ, et al. [Perioperative management of severe obstructive sleep apnea hypopnea syndrome]. Nan Fang Yi Ke Da Xue Xue Bao 2006;26(5):661–3 [in Chinese].

[31] Kim JA, Lee JJ. Preoperative predictors of difficult intubation in patients with obstructive sleep apnea syndrome. Can J Anaesth 2006;53(4):393–7.

[32] Wieczorek PM, Carli F. Obstructive sleep apnea uncovered after high spinal anesthesia: a case report. Can J Anaesth 2005;52(7):761–4.

[33] Kaw R, Michota F, Jaffer A, et al. Unrecognized sleep apnea in the surgical patient: implications for the perioperative setting. Chest 2006; 129(1):198–205.

[34] Onal E, Leech JA, Lopata M. Relationship between pulmonary-function and sleep-induced respiratory abnormalities. Chest 1985;87(4): 437–41.

[35] Boushra NN. Anaesthetic management of patients with sleep apnoea syndrome. Can J Anaesth 1996;43(6):599–616.

[36] Pelosi P, Croci M, Ravagnan I, et al. Total respiratory system, lung, and chest wall mechanics in sedated-paralyzed postoperative morbidly obese patients. Chest 1996;109(1):144–51.

[37] Sargent MA, McEachern AM, Jamieson DH, et al. Atelectasis on pediatric chest CT: comparison of sedation techniques. Pediatr Radiol 1999;29(7): 509–13.

[38] Catley DM, Thornton C, Jordan C, et al. Pronounced, episodic oxygen desaturation in the postoperative period—its association with ventilatory pattern and analgesic regimen. Anesthesiology 1985;63(1):20–8.

[39] Sollevi A, Lindahl SGE. Hypoxic and hypercapnic ventilatory responses during isoflurane sedation and anesthesia in women. Acta Anaesthesiol Scand 1995;39(7):931–8.

[40] Nishino T, Shirahata M, Yonezawa T, et al. Comparison of changes in the hypoglossal and the phrenic-nerve activity in response to increasing depth of anesthesia in cats. Anesthesiology 1984;60(1):19–24.

[41] Meoli AL, Rosen CL, Kristo D, et al. Upper airway management of the adult patient with obstructive sleep apnea in the perioperative period–avoiding complications. Sleep 2003;26(8): 1060–5.

[42] Jones JG, Sapsford DJ, Wheatley RG. Postoperative hypoxemia—mechanisms and time course. Anaesthesia 1990;45(7):566–73.

[43] Tierney NM, Pollard BJ, Doran BRH. Obstructive sleep-apnea. Anaesthesia 1989;44(3):235–7.

[44] Kavey NB, Altshuler KZ. Sleep in herniorrhaphy patients. Am J Surg 1979;138(5):682–7.

[45] Aurell J, Elmqvist D. Sleep in the surgical intensive-care unit—continuous polygraphic recording of sleep in 9 patients receiving postoperative care. BMJ 1985;290(6474):1029–32.

[46] Knill RL, Moote CA, Skinner MI, et al. Anesthesia with abdominal-surgery leads to intense REM-sleep during the 1st postoperative week. Anesthesiology 1990;73(1):52–61.

[47] Kehlet H, Rosenberg J. Late postoperative hypoxemia and organ dysfunction. Eur J Anaesthesiol 1995;12:31–4.

[48] Gupta RM, Parvizi J, Hanssen AD, et al. Postoperative complications in patients with obstructive sleep apnea syndrome undergoing hip or

knee replacement: a case-control study. Mayo Clin Proc 2001;76(9):897–905.

[49] Levin BC, Becker GD. Uvulopalatopharyngo-plasty for snoring—long-term results. Laryngoscope 1994;104(9):1150–2.

[50] Ben-Shlomo A, Melmed S. Clinical review 154: the role of pharmacotherapy in perioperative management of patients with acromegaly. J Clin Endocrinol Metab 2003;88(3):963–8.

[51] Donadio V, Liguori R, Vetrugno R, et al. Parallel changes in resting muscle sympathetic nerve activity and blood pressure in a hypertensive OSAS patient demonstrate treatment efficacy. Clin Auton Res 2006;16(3):235–9.

[52] Arzt M, Bradley TD. Treatment of sleep apnea in heart failure. Am J Respir Crit Care Med 2006; 173(12):1300–8.

[53] Winakur SJ, Smith PL, Schwartz AR. Pathophysiology and risk factors for obstructive sleep apnea. Semin Respir Crit Care Med 1998;19(2):99–112.

[54] Norman D, Loredo JS, Nelesen RA, et al. Effects of continuous positive airway pressure versus supplemental oxygen on 24-hour ambulatory blood pressure. Hypertension 2006;47(5):840–5.

[55] Robinson GV, Smith DM, Langford BA, et al. Continuous positive airway pressure does not reduce blood pressure in nonsleepy hypertensive OSA patients. Eur Respir J 2006;27(6):1229–35.

[56] Flemons WW, Whitelaw WA, Brant R, et al. Likelihood ratios for a sleep-apnea clinical-prediction rule. Am J Respir Crit Care Med 1994; 150(5):1279–85.

[57] Shivalkar B, Van de Heyning C, et al. Obstructive sleep apnea syndrome—more insights on structural and functional cardiac alterations, and the effects of treatment with continuous positive air-way pressure. J Am Coll Cardiol 2006; 47(7):1433–9.

[58] Czupryniak L, Loba J, Pawlowski M, et al. Treatment with continuous positive airway pressure may affect blood glucose levels in nondiabetic patients with obstructive sleep apnea syndrome. Sleep 2005;28(5):601–3.

[59] Ryan CF, Lowe AA, Li D, et al. Magnetic-resonance-imaging of the upper airway in obstructive sleep-apnea before and after chronic nasal continuous positive airway pressure therapy. Am Rev Respir Dis 1991;144(4):939–44.

[60] Pae EK, Lowe AA, Fleetham JA. A role of pharyngeal length in obstructive sleep apnea patients.

Am J Orthod Dentofacial Orthop 1997;111(1): 12–7.

[61] Ferretti A, Giampiccolo P, Cavalli A, et al. Expiratory flow limitation and orthopnea in massively obese subjects. Chest 2001;119(5):1401–8.

[62] Pawlik MT, Hansen E, Waldhauser D, et al. Clonidine premedication in patients with sleep apnea syndrome: a randomized, double-blind, placebo-controlled study. Anesth Analg 2005; 101(5):1374–80.

[63] American Society of Anesthesiologists. Practice guidelines for the perioperative management of patients with obstructive sleep apnea—a report by the Task Force on Perioperative Management of Patients with obstructive Sleep Apnea. Anesthesiology 2006;104(5):1081–93.

[64] Wilson PA, Skatrud JB, Dempsey JA. Effects of slow-wave sleep on ventilatory compensation to inspiratory elastic loading. Respir Physiol 1984;55(1):103–20.

[65] Wiegand L, Zwillich CW, White DP. Sleep and the ventilatory response to resistive loading in normal Men. J Appl Physiol 1988;64(3): 1186–95.

[66] Sjogren D, Sollevi A, Lindahl SGE. Isoflurane anesthesia and the ventilatory response to sustained isocapnic hypoxia in women. Anesthesiology 1995;83(3A):A1244.

[67] Eastwood PR, Szollosi I, Platt PR, et al. Comparison of upper airway collapse during general anaesthesia and sleep. Lancet 2002;359(9313): 1207–9.

[68] Gyulay S, Olson LG, Hensley MJ, et als NA. A comparison of clinical-assessment and home oximetry in the diagnosis of obstructive sleep-apnea. Am Rev Respir Dis 1993;147(1):50–3.

[69] Schafer H, Ewig S, Hasper E, et al. Predictive diagnostic value of clinical assessment and nonlaboratory monitoring system recordings in patients with symptoms suggestive of obstructive sleep apnea syndrome. Respiration (Herrlisheim) 1997;64(3):194–9.

[70] Tami TA, Duncan HJ, Pfleger M. Identification of obstructive sleep apnea in patients who snore. Laryngoscope 1998;108(4):508–13.

[71] Schellenberg JB, Maislin G, Schwab RJ. Physical findings and the risk for obstructive sleep apnea—the importance of oropharyngeal structures. Am J Respir Crit Care Med 2000;162(2): 740–8.

SLEEP
MEDICINE
CLINICS

Sleep Med Clin 1 (2007) 549–553

Index

Note: Page numbers of article titles are in **boldface** type.

A

Abdominal motion, in assessment of sleep-related breathing disorders, 452–454

Adherence, with positive airway pressure therapy. See Compliance, patient.

Airflow, assessment of, in sleep-related breathing disorders, 452

Analgesic agents, effect on respiratory system in patients with obstructive sleep apnea, 542

Anesthetics, effect on respiratory system in patients with obstructive sleep apnea, 542

Apnea, scoring of, in assessment of sleep-related breathing disorders, 457–458
See also Obstructive sleep apnea syndrome.

Appliances, oral, impact on quality of life in patients with obstructive sleep apnea, 522
in treatment for upper airway respiratory syndrome, 480

Architecture, sleep, in upper airway resistance syndrome, 476

Arousals, respiratory effort-related, scoring of, in assessment of sleep-related breathing disorders, 459

Assessment, of sleep-related breathing disorders, **449–460, 461–463**
clinical, **449–460**
interviews, 449–450, 451, 452
questionnaires, 450, 453, 454
laboratory, with polysomnography, **449–460**
interpretation, 460
recording, 450–456
scoring, 456–460
nonlaboratory, **461–463**
cardiopulmonary recorder assessment, 462
interpretation and disposition, 462–463
pretest clinical assessment, 461–462

Asthma, nocturnal, in differential diagnosis of upper airway resistance syndrome, 479

Automated scoring, of cyclic alternating pattern (CAP), **483–489**
development of, 484–485
translational research using, 486–488
vs. visual scoring, validation of, 485–486

Autotitrating positive airway pressure (APAP), for obstructive sleep apnea, 530

B

Breathing disorders, sleep-related, **443–548**
assessment of, **449–460, 461–463**
clinical, **449–460**
interview, 449–450, 451, 452
questionnaires, 450, 453, 454
laboratory, with polysomnography, **449–460**
interpretation, 460
recording, 450–456
scoring, 456–460
nonlaboratory, **461–463**
cardiopulmonary recorder assessment, 462
interpretation and disposition, 462–463
pretest clinical assessment, 461–462
cyclic alternating pattern (CAP) and, **483–489**
automated *vs.* visual scoring, validation of, 485–486
definition of, 483–484
development of scoring for, 484–485
translational research in, 486–488
epidemiology of, **443–447**
comorbidities, 445–446
data comparisons, 445–446
Veterans Health Administration databases, 444–445
home monitoring, economics of, **465–473**
mood disorders and, **513–517**
discussion, 516–517
methods of study on, 514–515

doi:10.1016/S1556-407X(07)00013-6

Moving?

Make sure your subscription moves with you!

To notify us of your new address, find your **Clinics Account Number** (located on your mailing label above your name), and contact customer service at:

E-mail: elspcs@elsevier.com

800-654-2452 (subscribers in the U.S. & Canada)
407-345-4000 (subscribers outside of the U.S. & Canada)

Fax number: 407-363-9661

Elsevier Periodicals Customer Service
6277 Sea Harbor Drive
Orlando, FL 32887-4800

*To ensure uninterrupted delivery of your subscription, please notify us at least 4 weeks in advance of move.

ELSEVIER